SAMUEL BAVLI

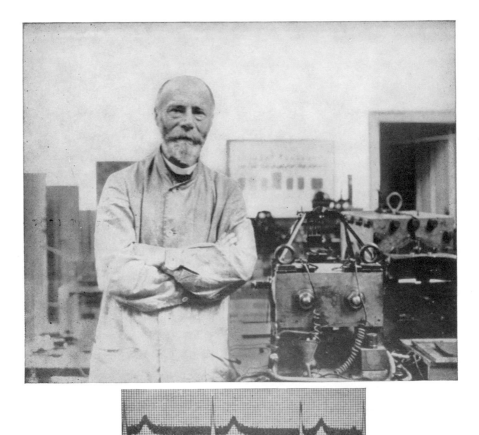

WILLEM EINTHOVEN AND HIS ORIGINAL GALVANOMETER IN HIS
LABORATORY. A RECORD MADE WITH THIS GALVANOMETER.
(Courtesy, Cambridge Instrument Co., New York)

A Primer of
Electrocardiography

GEORGE E. BURCH, M.D., F.A.C.P., F.A.C.C.

*Henderson Professor of Medicine, Tulane University Echool of Medicine; Physician-
in-Chief, Tulane Unit. Charity Hospital; Consultant in Cardiovascular Diseases,
Ochsner Clinic, Ochsner Foundation Hospital, Veterans Administration
Hospital; Consultant in Medicine, Hotel Dieu, Illinois Central Hospital,
Touro Infirmary, U. S. Public Health Service Hospital, New Orleans*

TRAVIS WINSOR, M.D., F.A.C.P.

*Associate Clinical Professor of Medicine, University of Southern California,
School of Medicine; Director, Wiley Winsor Memorial Heart Research
Foundation; Staff Member, St. Vincent's Hospital, The Hospital of
the Good Samaritan and the Los Angeles County General
Hospital, Los Angeles*

Fifth Edition

286 Illustrations

LEA & FEBIGER

PHILADELPHIA   1966

First Edition, 1945

Reprinted, 1945, 1946 (3 times), 1947 (twice), and 1948
French Edition, 1948
Spanish Edition, 1948
Czechoslovakia, 1948

Second Edition, 1949

Reprinted, 1949, (twice), 1950, 1951, 1953, and 1954
French Edition, 1954
Spanish Edition, 1951

Third Edition, 1955

Reprinted, 1955, 1956, and 1958
Italian Edition, 1958
Serbo-Croat Edition, 1958
Spanish Edition, 1958

Fourth Edition, 1960

Reprinted, 1961 and 1963
Greek Edition, 1961
Japanese Edition, 1961
Spanish Edition, 1964

Fifth Edition, 1966

Library of Congress Catalog Card Number: 66–19291

Printed in The United States of America

Dedicated

TO

Vivian Gerard Burch

AND

Elizabeth Adams Winsor

WITH GRATITUDE AND APPRECIATION FOR THEIR INESTIMABLE
ASSISTANCE AND ENCOURAGEMENT IN ALL OF OUR ENDEAVORS

PREFACE TO THE FIFTH EDITION

THIS book apparently has been successfully serving an educational purpose. It is intended for beginners. It is not encyclopedic, but rather presents fundamental principles and concepts of electrocardiography. Once the beginner has reached a more advanced stage of training, the literature and experience will provide opportunities for more advanced training. With these objectives in mind it was considered advisable to alter the book only slightly. There have been no great changes in the concepts of electrocardiography within the last six years to justify any marked changes in this book. The fundamentals of vectorcardiography have not advanced sufficiently to require changes in this field. Until a simple, reliable and reproducible reference frame of electrode placement is agreed upon for the world, vectorcardiography cannot serve physicians sufficiently to justify its clinical use. Furthermore, vectorcardiography must be shown to add enough to clinical electrocardiography to justify routine use and to make it recommendable to practicing physicians. For such reasons, the discussions on vectorcardiography were not expanded.

In the discussions of the electrocardiograph, adherence to the string galvanometer was deemed advisable because the presentation provides fundamental concepts of the functions and principles of any galvanometer. Once these principles are understood, the student should have relatively little difficulty translating them to the direct writing galvanometer, cathode ray oscilloscope or any other type of recorder. Furthermore, the clinical reliability of the string galvanometer cannot be overemphasized.

The tables in the appendix are modified to include more data on normal values for infants, children and adults. The role of the electrocardiogram in the diagnosis of infarction of areas of the myocardium which are depolarized late or during mid-temporal periods of the cardiac electric cycle is emphasized further. The electrocardiographic diagnostic criteria for papillary muscle infarction are discussed. Minor corrections and modifications were made as indicated.

We wish to thank Miss Juanita Arbour and Miss Ruth Ziifle for their unselfish interest and excellent editorial assistance in the preparation of this edition. The usual fine and friendly assistance and cooperation of Lea & Febiger is gratefully acknowledged. It is hoped that this book will continue to serve a useful purpose in clinical medicine.

New Orleans, Louisiana   G. E. B.
Los Angeles, California   T. W.

PREFACE TO THE FIRST EDITION

THIS primer was written to enable the student who is unfamiliar with the subject to grasp a fundamental knowledge of electrocardiography in the most direct manner. Although no photographs of electrocardiograms are included, diagrams are liberally employed to illustrate typical electrocardiographic patterns and to depict certain conceptions more clearly. Obviously, this primer is a supplement to the many monographs on electrocardiography that are now available and which should be consulted and used in conjunction with it.

While this book is necessarily somewhat dogmatic, we think a certain amount of dogmatism is essential for the proper introduction to, and a clear understanding of, such a subject as electrocardiography. Certain concepts of a special nature are eliminated, not because they are deemed unimportant but in order to keep this presentation simple and brief. Further study of the subject is necessary before one should be permitted to undertake the serious responsibility of reading electrocardiograms clinically, and it is hoped that the student's interest will be aroused to such an extent that he will continue with more detailed study of the problem. This primer is only the foundation upon which to build a useful, practical and theoretical knowledge of electrocardiography.

Within the scope of this presentation it is impossible to discuss the anatomy, physiology and pharmacology of the heart, and it is assumed that the reader possesses information on these subjects. The student should provide himself with such necessary information before he undertakes the study of electrocardiography.

Material has been drawn freely from the literature, particularly from the publications of Dr. Richard Ashman and Dr. Frank Wilson and their co-workers. We wish to express our indebtedness and appreciation to these authors. With rare exceptions, bibliographic references have been omitted, since the nature of this primer does not warrant the inclusion of a full bibliography.

The authors are grateful to Dr. J. H. Musser, Professor of Medicine at Tulane University School of Medicine, for his suggestions and encouragement during the development of the work. Indebtedness is acknowledged to Drs. R. H. Bayley and J. M. Bamber for their helpful criticisms. Gratitude is also expressed to Miss Vera Morel, who made the drawings, and to Mrs. Gusse Patten for her editorial assistance.

G. E. B.

New Orleans, Louisiana   T. W.

CONTENTS

CHAPTER 1

PRINCIPLES OF ELECTROCARDIOGRAPHY

CHAPTER 2

AN ANALYSIS OF VARIOUS COMPONENTS OF THE ELECTROCARDIOGRAM AND THEIR CLINICAL SIGNIFICANCE

CHAPTER 3

PRECORDIAL LEADS

Contents

CHAPTER 4

DISORDERS OF THE HEART BEAT

CHAPTER 5

CLINICAL APPLICATIONS OF THE ELECTROCARDIOGRAM

Contents

APPENDIX

Chapter 1

PRINCIPLES OF ELECTROCARDIOGRAPHY

THE ELECTROCARDIOGRAPH

I⊤ has been known for many years that a measurable amount of electric current is associated with activity of the heart. Ludwig and Waller, in 1887, experimented with the capillary electroscope and recorded this electromotive force from the precordium. Einthoven's description, in 1903, of the string galvanometer, a sensitive and quantitative instrument, stimulated a sudden increase in both clinical and experimental studies of electrocardiography. This type of galvanometer has remained one of the most useful, although other principles, such as the use of vacuum tube amplification, have been applied. In fact, the best fidelity is obtained with vacuum tube amplifiers and cathode-ray oscilloscopic recording. Because of simplicity and portability, direct writing electrocardiographs are used almost exclusively today by doctors in practice.

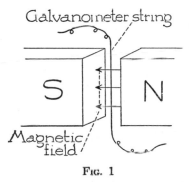

FIG. 1

The *string galvanometer* consists of a strong electromagnet, between the poles of which is suspended a string made of a quartz glass fiber about the diameter of an erythrocyte (7.8μ). The fiber is coated with platinum or silver to permit the transmission of an electric current (Fig. 1).

The *magnetic field* is a field of constant force set up by a strong fixed magnet or electromagnet. The force always runs from the North (N) to the South (S) pole of the magnet. Current from the heart, conducted through the string, creates another magnetic field of force which runs around the long axis of the string and travels either in a clockwise or counterclockwise direction as viewed from an end of the string, depending

2

upon the direction of flow of current in the string. This field coursing around the string is a *magnetic field of variable force*, the magnitude of which depends upon the magnitude of the current flowing through the string. It is the interaction of these two magnetic fields with each other that causes movement of the string.

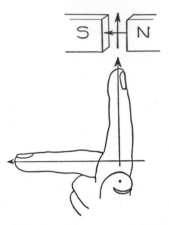

FIG. 2.—Direction of string deflection. The arrows indicate the direction of action of the various forces. (See text for details.)

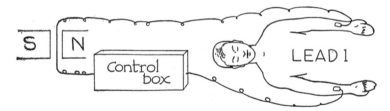

FIG. 3A.—A schematic representation of connections for lead I and a diagram of the optical system.

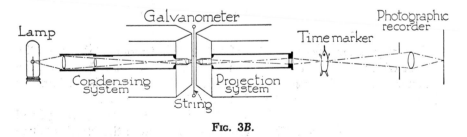

FIG. 3B.

Two practical working rules for predicting the movement of the string in any instance are the right hand rules, the first of which, (1) Ampere's rule, states that if the string is grasped by the right hand and the thumb points in the direction of the current of flow, the fingers grasping the string will point in the direction of the electromagnetic field; the second of which, (2) a modification of Fleming's rule, states that if the thumb and index finger are held extended in the same plane as the palm, the middle finger is flexed to make a 90 degree angle with the palm, the index finger is pointed in the direction of flow of current in the string, and the middle finger is pointed in the direction of the magnetic field, the thumb then will indicate the direction in which the string will move. In figure 2 the current is flowing upward in the string, and the deflection of the string is toward the reader. If the current were flowing downward in the string, the deflection would be away from the reader.

In order to record an electrocardiogram, one terminus of the string is connected to the right arm (RA) and the other is connected to the left arm (LA) of the subject. Electrodes properly connected to these parts constitute *lead I* (Fig. 3A). Other leads may be recorded by connecting the electrodes to different parts of the body (see p. 31).

The control box consists of a small dry cell battery and a series of resistors which make it possible to balance "currents of injury," skin currents and other extraneous currents as well as to standardize the sensitivity of the string.

By means of a system of lenses similar to those used in a microscope, the shadow of the quartz string is focused on the slit of a camera in which photographic paper moves. This makes it possible to record the deflections of the string (Fig. 3B). The finished record is known as the *electrocardiogram*.

THE NORMAL ELECTROCARDIOGRAM

The typical electrocardiogram of a cardiac cycle, represented diagrammatically in figure 4, consists of a series of waves arbitrarily designated by Einthoven as the *P wave*, the *QRS complex*, the *T wave* and the *U wave*. Normal values of magnitude and duration for these waves are in the Appendix (Tables 2 to 6).

It is well to note that the electromotive force (EMF) that is responsible for the P wave and the QRS complex occurs *before the auricular and ventricular muscle fibers contract* and not as a result of their contraction.

The P Wave.—The width of the P wave, measured in seconds from the beginning to the end of the wave, does not normally exceed 0.11 second. The height of the normal wave in any lead does not usually exceed 2.5 millimeters (Fig. 5 and Appendix, Table 2).

The P wave represents the depolarization wave of the auricular musculature which spreads radially from the sinoauricular (SA) node to the atrioventricular (AV) node.

The P–R Segment.—There is a delay in transmission of the impulse at the AV node, represented on the electrocardiogram by the P–R segment. The auricular T wave (see p. 80), the repolarization wave of

the auricles, is usually contained in this segment and in the QRS complex.
The P–R segment is measured in seconds from the end of the P wave to
the beginning of the QRS complex (Fig. 4).

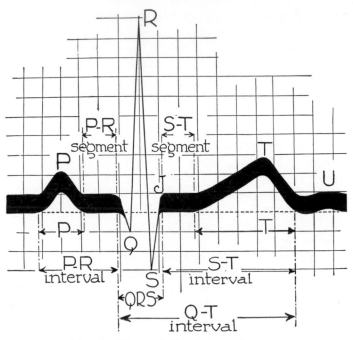

FIG. 4.—Waves of the electrocardiogram.

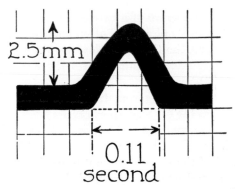

FIG. 5.—P wave and its measurements. The greatest amplitude is usually
seen in lead II.

The P–R Interval.—The P–R interval is measured from the beginning
of the P wave to the beginning of the QRS complex. If the ventricular
(QRS) complex begins with an initial downward deflection, the Q wave,
then the interval is sometimes spoken of as the P–Q interval. The P–R

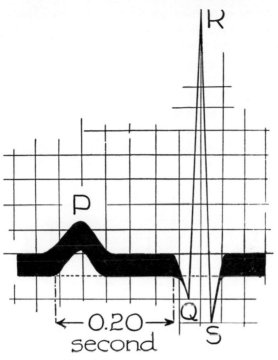

FIG. 6.—The P–R interval and the upper limit of normal for cardiac rates of 70–90 beats per minute in adults.

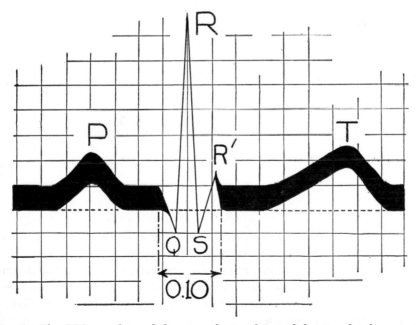

FIG. 7.—The QRS complex and the upper limits of normal duration for the average normal cardiac rate (70–90 per minute).

or P–Q interval represents the time required to depolarize the atrial musculature plus the delay in transmission of the impulse through the atrioventricular node to the beginning of ventricular depolarization. The
upper limit of normal for the duration of the P–R (or P–Q) interval for
average cardiac rates in adults (70–90) is 0.20 second (Fig. 6 and
Appendix, Table 3).

The QRS Complex.—The QRS complex is the depolarization complex
of the ventricular musculature. It consists, usually, of an initial downward deflection, the *Q wave*, an initial upward deflection, the *R wave*, the
initial downward deflection after the R wave, the *S wave*, and a second

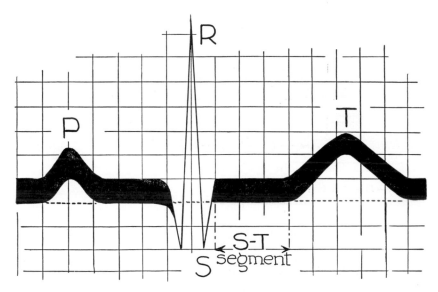

FIG. 8.—The duration of the S–T segment (duration of the depolarized state) varies
greatly with the cardiac rate.

upward deflection, the second positive deflection or the *R prime* (*R'*)
wave. The duration of the QRS interval is measured in seconds from the
beginning of the first wave of the complex to the end of the last wave and,
for practical purposes, does not exceed 0.10 second normally (Fig. 7 and
Appendix, Table 4).

The S-T Segment.—That portion of the electrocardiogram between the
end of the QRS complex and the beginning of the T wave is known as the
S–T segment. It represents, roughly, the depolarized state, or the duration
of the *excited state* of the ventricular musculature, or the interval of time
between the completion of depolarization and the beginning of repolarization of the ventricular musculature (Fig. 8). The variations are shown
in the Appendix (Table 5).

Principles of Electrocardiography

23

The S–T Interval.—The duration in seconds from the end of the QRS complex to the end of the T wave is known as the *S–T interval*. It represents the time from completion of depolarization of the ventricular musculature to completion of repolarization (Fig. 9).

The Junction, J.—The point of junction between the QRS complex and the S–T segment is known as the Junction, J (Fig. 10).

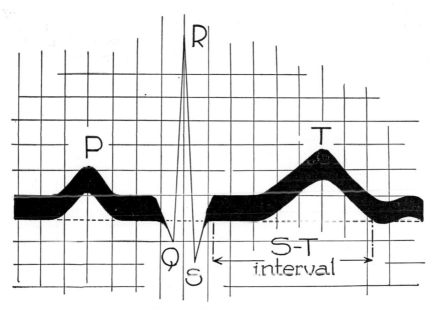

FIG. 9.—The S–T interval.

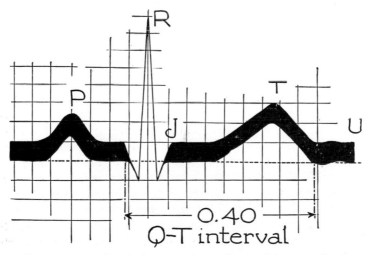

FIG. 10.—The Q–T interval with the upper limit of normal for a cardiac rate of 70.

The Q–T Interval.—This interval is measured in seconds from the beginning of the QRS complex to the end of the T wave (Fig. 10) and represents the entire time required for depolarization and repolarization of the ventricular musculature. It varies with age, sex, and cardiac rate (see Table 6 in the Appendix). The upper limit of normal for a cardiac rate of 70 is 0.40 second.

The T Wave.—The T wave is the wave of ventricular repolarization (Fig. 10). Its amplitude and duration vary considerably, as indicated by Table 2 of the Appendix. The T wave will be discussed in detail later.

The U Wave.—The U wave is an "after-potential" wave which follows the T wave and is usually low in amplitude (Figs. 4 and 10).

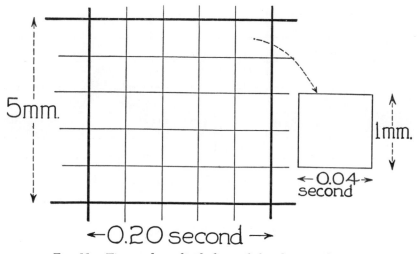

FIG. 11.—Time and amplitude lines of the electrocardiogram.

THE TIME AND MILLIMETER LINES OF THE ELECTROCARDIOGRAM

Horizontal and vertical lines are inscribed on the electrocardiogram. The former are 1 millimeter apart and represent 0.1 millivolt (100 microvolts) when the electrocardiogram is properly standardized. The vertical lines are time lines, separated from each other by an interval of 0.04 second. It is therefore customary to speak of the *duration* of the various segments, intervals and waves in seconds and of the *amplitude* in millimeters or millivolts. When the heart produces sufficient electromotive force (EMF) to cause a deflection of the string of 10 millimeters, the force involved is 1 millivolt. This is true only if the tension of the string is adjusted by the process of *standardization,* so that when 1 millivolt is added to or removed from the circuit, the string is deflected 10 millimeters.

For facility in measuring, every fifth vertical and horizontal line is wider than the others. The distance between two adjacent wide vertical lines represents 0.20 second and the distance between the two adjacent wide horizontal lines represents 5 millimeters (Fig. 11).

BASES OF THE THEORY OF ELECTROCARDIOGRAPHY

The present concept of the theory of electrocardiography is based upon data collected from many sources. Some of the main sources of information are:

1. Clinical data collected on patients during life and correlated with information found at necropsy.

2. Physiologic observations on the intact hearts of experimental animals, such as the frog, turtle, dog, cat, and other animals.

3. Study of isolated muscle strips.

4. Studies on the *giant axon of the squid*, as well as observations made on other nerves by neurophysiologists.

5. Studies on the large one cell plant, such as the *Nitella flexilis*. This cell, like the giant axon of the squid, lends itself well to the study of depolarization and repolarization processes. An electrode can be inserted into this relatively large structure with ease, and another may be placed upon the surface or in a medium bathing it.

THE VOLUME CONDUCTOR

A *volume conductor* is a medium which permits the conduction of electricity in three dimensions. A good example is a large vessel containing physiologic saline solution or any type of ions in water. In figure 12 is shown a glass tank containing physiologic saline solution, a volume conductor. *The human body*, by virtue of the chemical nature of its fluids, is essentially a volume conductor, its boundary being limited by the body surface. Thus, current generated in any part of the body can reach any other part.

Current may be caused to flow in the volume conductor if two electrodes which are insulated except for their tips, are inserted into the saline bath and their opposite ends are connected to the poles of a battery (Fig. 13).

A positive electric field of force will exist around one electrode, the *anode*, and a negative field around the other, the *cathode*. These fields may be detected and their extent may be mapped out by use of a galvanometer connected to a fixed distant or "indifferent" electrode (p) and a movable "exploring" electrode (P). The former is placed at a distant point in the volume conductor, so that the electric fields produced by the battery influence it little or, for practical purposes, not at all. The exploring electrode is moved about in the vicinity of the electrodes from

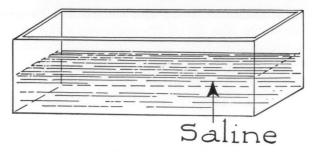

Saline

FIG. 12.—A volume conductor.

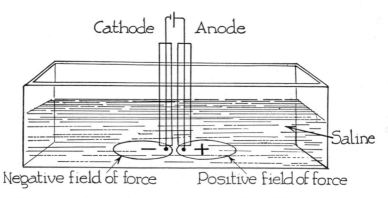

Cathode   Anode

Saline

Negative field of force   Positive field of force

FIG. 13.—A volume conductor with copper electrodes and battery in place, indicating the positive and negative fields of force in one plane. The wires are heavily insulated except for their termini.

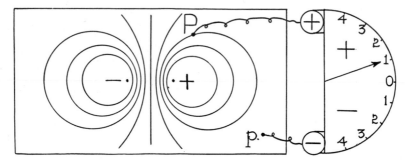

FIG. 14.—Volume conductor and tips of copper anode and cathode shown in figure 13 viewed from below. The galvanometer connected to an indifferent electrode (*p*) and to an exploring electrode (*P*) is used to map out the electric fields of force about the anode and cathode.*

*In figure 14 and all similar figures to follow, the + and − signs in the circles on the galvanometer represent binding posts. When current flows through the galvanometer from the positive binding post to the negative one, the galvanometer deflects in the positive direction. Thus, when a point within a system under study is relatively positive with respect to another point in the system and the former is connected to the positive binding post, a positive deflection in the galvanometer follows.

the battery (Fig. 14) in order to map out the fields of potential about the anode and cathode.

If the exploring electrode is placed near the positive pole, a positive or upward deflection (Fig. 14) of the galvanometer needle results, and if the exploring electrode is placed near the negative pole, a negative or downward deflection of the galvanometer needle will take place. The *fixed* or *"indifferent" electrode* is placed so far from the origin of the field

Isopotential lines

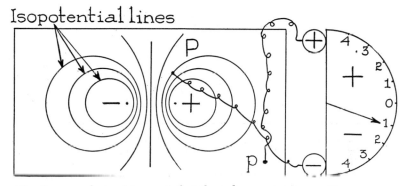

Fig. 15.—Same as figure 14 except that the galvanometer connections are reversed, thus deflecting the needle to the negative side of the galvanometer.

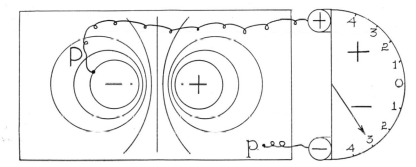

Fig. 16.—The exploring electrode is in a field of relative negativity and a downward or negative deflection of the needle or string results.

of force that when the *exploring electrode* is placed close to the source of the respective forces, a great influence is exerted on the latter electrode. As the electrode is moved away, the force decreases by the square of the distance moved. It is this inequality of influences on the two electrodes that produces electric differences (an EMF), a flow of current resulting, which in turn deflects the string or needle of the galvanometer.

Obviously, if the electrode connections to the galvanometer are switched so that the exploring electrode is attached to the negative instead of the positive terminal of the galvanometer and the indifferent electrode is placed on the positive terminal, then the needle of the galvanometer will reverse its direction of movement when the exploring electrode is now placed in the respective electric fields described in the preceding paragraph (Fig. 15). In other words, it is possible to vary the direction of movement of the galvanometer needle by varying the connections to the galvanometer.

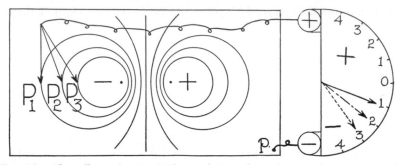

Fig. 17.—The effect of moving the exploring electrode (P) from the periphery toward the negative pole of the doublet on the deflection of the galvanometer needle. P is successively placed on three different isopotential lines, P_1, P_2, and P_3. The following examples illustrate the increase of force which results as the exploring electrode is moved closer to the negative pole of the doublet.

The difference in potential is the algebraic difference between the electric potential at P and p. Thus, $P–p$ is equal to the potential difference. The force acting at p is essentially 0. The force acting at P_1 is negative and is equal to 1 unit, at P_2 it is negative and equal to 2 units, and at P_3 it is negative and exerts a force equal to 3 units. The differences in potentials therefore are respectively:

Example 1: $-1-0=-1$ unit of electric potential.
Example 2: $-2-0=-2$ units of electric potential.
Example 3: $-3-0=-3$ units of electric potential.

Thus, in all examples the direction is negative, and the potential increases as the exploring electrode approaches the negative pole of the dipole.

It is well to remember that within the organism the current flows from the point of more negative potential to the point of more positive potential, whereas in the galvanometer it flows from the point of more positive potential to the point of more negative potential (Fig. 18).

When the exploring electrode is near the positive pole or anode, it is in a "*field of positivity*" and is considered to be in a "*field of relative positivity*," i.e., relatively positive when compared with the indifferent electrode, which is at a weakly positive potential. This results in a deflection of the galvanometer needle to the positive direction (Fig. 14). When the exploring electrode is brought near the negative pole or cathode, it is in a "*field of negativity*" and is also in a "*field of relative negativity*" when compared with the indifferent electrode. The latter results in a deflection of the galvanometer needle to the negative direction (Fig. 16). A positive field of two units of potential, although of absolute positivity, is relatively negative when compared with a field of three units of positive potential.

The exposed copper terminals of the anode and cathode in the volume conductor, as shown in figures 13, 14, 15 and 16, constitute a doublet or dipole. One is the positive charge of the doublet and the other the negative charge. As the exploring electrode is moved around these negative points of the doublet, equipotential or isopotential lines can be mapped out (Fig. 17). The magnitude of the electric potential is the same at any point on an isopotential line. The electric force decreases as the exploring electrode is moved from the source of the respective charges and obeys the law:

$$\text{Electric Potential} \propto \frac{1}{d^2}, \text{ where } d = \text{unit of distance}$$

THE PATIENT AS A VOLUME CONDUCTOR

If we consider *the patient as a volume conductor* and the electric impulses originating in the heart as a source of potential differences, the magnitude and direction of the current produced may be measured.

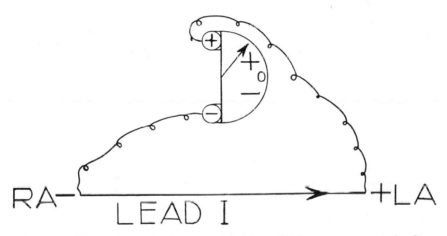

Fig. 18.—The arrow running between the right and left arms represents the direction of flow of current in the patient. In the galvanometer circuit the current flows from positive to negative field.

Lead I.—If a galvanometer, *the electrocardiograph*, is attached to the right and left arms of an individual, just above the wrists, the difference in potential between these points may be measured and recorded as lead I of the electrocardiogram. By arbitrary construction of the electrocardiograph, the current is conducted intentionally through the galvanometer so that whenever the right arm is relatively negative and the left arm is relatively positive, there is recorded an upward or positive deflection on the completed electrocardiogram (Fig. 18).

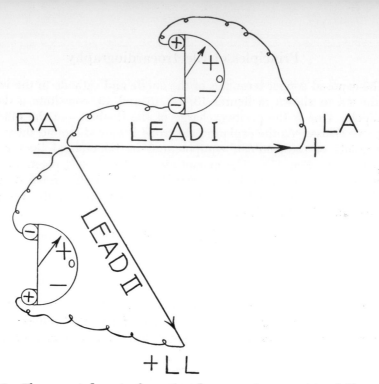

RA LEAD I LA

LEAD II

+LL

FIG. 19.—The current flows in the patient from negative to positive field. In the galvanometer it flows from positive to negative field.

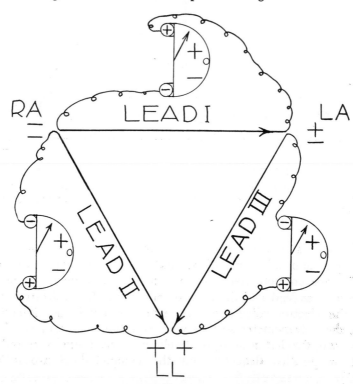

RA LEAD I LA

LEAD II LEAD III

++
LL

FIG. 20.—Leads I, II and III *(Standard leads or limb leads)*. Current flowing in directions as indicated by the arrows produces upright deflections for each of these three leads.

Lead II.—The electrodes are attached to the right arm above the wrist and to the left leg just above the ankle to record lead II. The current is conducted through the galvanometer in such a manner as to produce an upward or positive deflection in the finished electrocardiogram whenever the right arm is relatively negative and the left leg relatively positive (Fig. 19).

Lead III.—The electrodes are attached to the left arm and left leg to record lead III. The current is conducted through the galvanometer in such a manner as to produce an upward or positive deflection in the finished electrocardiogram whenever the left arm is relatively negative and the left leg relatively positive.

These three leads together constitute the standard or limb leads (Fig. 20).

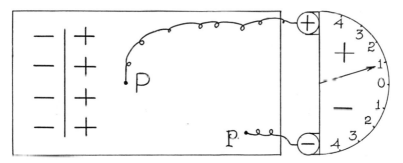

Fig. 21.—A polarized membrane.

THE POLARIZED (RESTING) STATE, DEPOLARIZATION, THE DEPOLARIZED (EXCITED) STATE, AND REPOLARIZATION

The Polarized State.—In previous figures doublets were shown. Living resting cells have a series of such doublets along their walls, the positive charge being along the external surface and the negative charge along the internal surface. When these doublets are located around the surface of the cell, the cell membrane is said to be *polarized*. A polarized membrane is shown in a volume conductor in figure 21, and a polarized living resting cell is shown in figure 22. Metabolic processes, processes of life, are necessary to maintain the polarized state.

The electric forces about *a single polarized membrane* may be studied with a galvanometer and indifferent and exploring electrodes. The deflection of the needle of the galvanometer will be either negative or positive (Fig. 21), depending upon the proximity of the exploring electrode to the negative or positive charges on the polarized membrane. The *amplitude* of the deflection depends upon the magnitude of the acting electric force, and the *direction* depends upon the direction of flow of the current in the galvanometer. When the exploring (*P*) and the indifferent

(p) electrodes are equidistant from the opposite surface of the membrane (Fig. 23), twice as much current flows as when the indifferent (p) is at a great distance from the membrane.

The magnitude of the electromotive force exerted by the charges on the membrane at the point P can be expressed in the following manner: If, from the point P, lines are extended to the edges of the membrane, a *solid angle* will be formed at P. If the membrane is a spherical cell, a cone will

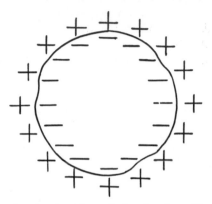

FIG. 22.—A normal resting cell showing its wall polarized.

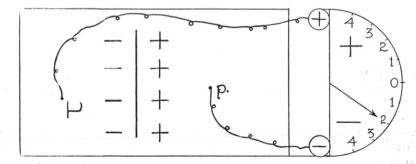

FIG 23.—The EMF represents the difference in potential between the force acting at P and p. For example, if -1 unit of force is acting at P and $+1$ unit of force is acting at p, the algebraic difference is $-$ P $-$ ($+ p$) or $-1 - (+1)$ or -2. The deflection of the string is negative and the EMF is 2 units, so that the galvanometer registers -2.

be produced by the lines extending from P. Although three-dimensional, this cone is represented graphically (Fig. 24) as existing in one plane only.

If a sphere of unit area is then described about the point P, *the area on the surface of the sphere cut off by the cone* will be proportional to the magnitude of the potential exerted by the charges on the membrane at the point p (Fig. 25).

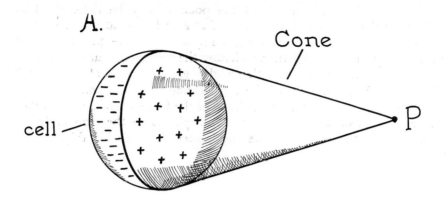

A.

Cone

cell

P

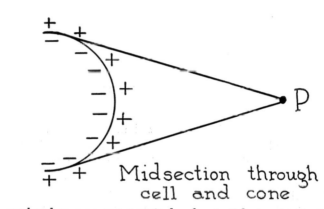

B.

Midsection through
cell and cone

FIG. 24.—A.   Cone employed to represent magnitude of potential at point *P*.   *B*.
Midsection through cone shown in *A*. For simplicity, in all illustrations to follow
in this compendium, only midsections through the cone will be represented.

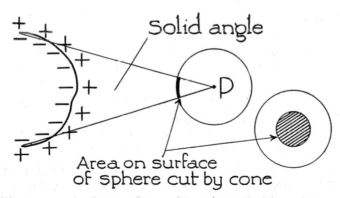

Solid angle

P

Area on surface
of cone cut by cone

FIG. 25—Manner of indicating force acting at point *P*. (See text for details.)

3

The effective charge acting at the point P may be determined as follows: If the observer stations himself at P and looks at the membrane or cell through a small hole made at the apex of the cone, the charge that meets his eye first will determine whether the force acting at P is positive or negative. Since the size of the solid angle subtended at the point P determines the magnitude of the force acting at P, the contour of the membrane will not alter the magnitude of the force or its sign (Fig. 26). The areas cut from the surface of the unit spheres are the same in figures 25 and 26, but the contours of the membranes differ considerably.

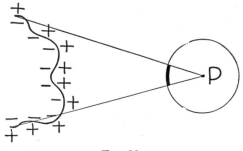

FIG. 26.

Depolarization.—Two polarized membranes A and B may be placed close together to form a sphere, a polarized "cell" (Fig. 27a). If the exploring electrode is placed at the point P and the indifferent electrode at a distant point in the volume conductor, there will be no flow of current, since there is no difference in potential between these two points. If a stimulus is applied to the "cell" at the point indicated by the arrow in figure 27a, there results a breakdown in the dielectric effect or resistance offered by the cell membrane to the migration together of the positive and negative charges. The negative charge migrates out and discharges the positive charge on the external surface of the "cell." In so doing, it reduces the resistance of the membrane in the immediate vicinity so that adjacent *doublets* are discharged, and these in turn lower the resistance locally, which allows the immediately adjacent doublets to become discharged. These phenomena continue successively until almost all the doublets of the entire cell are "discharged." This process of discharging the doublets is known as the process of *depolarization*, and the cell is said to be *depolarized*, or in the "excited state," when it is discharged (Fig. 27e). From figure 27 it can be seen that as this process progresses at a steady or equally rapid rate around the surface of the cell, a difference in potential is created between the points P and p in the volume conductor. If a record of this is made with a galvanometer, a curve or wave, known as the *wave of depolarization*, is inscribed.

Repolarization.—Immediately following depolarization of the cell, and during the period of contraction, if this be a muscle cell, certain "reparative" physicochemical processes begin to take place. After a short period of time, these processes result in restitution of the positive and negative charges to their respective positions along the surface of the membrane. This process of adding dipoles, known as *repolarization,* begins, under

DEPOLARIZATION PROCESS

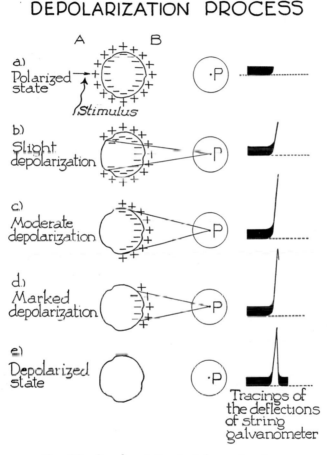

FIG. 27.—See descriptive text for explanation.

the conditions described, at those points where depolarization first began, since time is an important factor in the physicochemical changes leading up to repolarization. Furthermore, the repolarization process is associated with a difference in potential between the points P and p in the volume conductor (Fig. 28). Obviously, the wave recorded in this process, which is known as the *wave of repolarization,* will be in the opposite direction.

Since repolarization is slower than depolarization, the wave of the former does not fall and rise as abruptly as that of the latter. Furthermore, the repolarization process is actually "patchy" in appearance, so that the difference in potential at any one moment between points

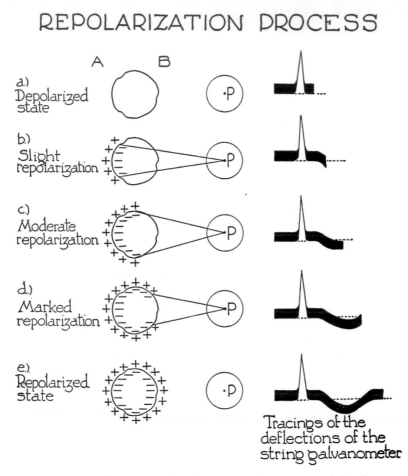

REPOLARIZATION PROCESS

A   B

a.) Depolarized state

b.) Slight repolarization

c.) Moderate repolarization

d.) Marked repolarization

e.) Repolarized state

Tracings of the deflections of the string galvanometer

FIG. 28.—Steps in the process of repolarization and inscription of the electrocardiogram. Repolarization begins where stimulation was applied and spreads progressively over the membranes. The recorded wave is negative in this instance.

P and p during repolarization is usually not as great as during depolarization, and the amplitude of the repolarization wave is, therefore, not as great as that of the depolarization wave. The area included under each wave is the same, for the total quantity of current involved in each process is the same. Since repolarization is active for a long period of time, its wave is of long duration although of low amplitude (Fig. 29).

It is well to note here that it is unkown how completely a membrane is depolarized when it is activated by a stimulus. Although it is shown for convenience in the accompanying diagrams to be completely depolarized, this is most probably not true, the process of depolarization being associated with only partial discharge of the doublets.°

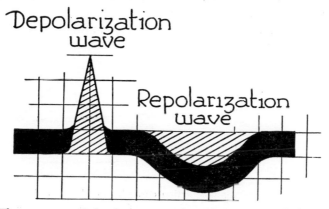

FIG. 29.—The processes of depolarization and repolarization result in two separate waves which include equal areas.

EFFECTS OF TEMPERATURE ON DEPOLARIZATION AND REPOLARIZATION

Since all these processes are associated with physicochemical phenomena, temperature has a definite effect upon them. It is well known that application of heat will increase the rate of chemical reactions and that removal of heat or cooling will retard the rate of such reactions. If we now cool only membrane B to 1° C. (Fig. 30) and then stimulate mem-

°The studies of Curtis and Cole and of Hodgkin indicate that when the wave of depolarization migrates over the surface of a cell, this process is not accompanied by a discharge of the positive and negative charges, as indicated previously. Instead, it is associated with a reversal of polarity along the surface of the membrane, i.e., the positive charges migrate to the internal aspect of the cell membrane and the negative charges to the external surface. With repolarization, the doublets again revert to the resting state, with the positive charges on the outside and negative ones on the inside. Although this concept is generally accepted, it is considered advisable to adhere to the ideas of depolarization and repolarization for simplicity of illustration and presentation, especially since the theoretic considerations remain unchanged except for the magnitude of the potential changes concerned with the electric activity of the cells. Furthermore, the concepts of depolarization and repolarization are easier for the student to visualize; once he has mastered the fundamental ideas, it is not difficult to grasp the ideas of Curtis and Cole. It is well to note that many observers refer to the waves of depolarization as waves of "accession" or "excitation" and the waves of repolarization as waves of "regression" or "recovery," all of which terms are noncommittal as to the exact nature of the underlying electric phenomena. Associated with depolarization, K leaves the cells and Na enters, whereas with repolarization, K returns to the cells and Na escapes to the extracellular space. The mechanisms for this shift and its relationship to the bioelectric phenomena remain unknown.

brane A at the point indicated by the arrow, only membrane A will be depolarized and repolarized, since the chemical processes along the surface of membrane B will be inhibited by the low temperature of 1° C. Membrane A will undergo the same changes as described in figures 27 and 28. This will produce a record or curve such as that in figure 30, produced by the *monophasic action current.* In this instance the record is a wave of a *positive monophasic action current.*

If membrane A is cooled to 1° C. and membrane B is stimulated, a *negative monophasic action current* results (Fig. 31).

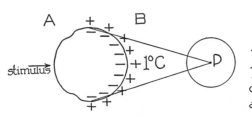
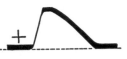

Resultant tracing is that of a positive monophasic action current

FIG. 30.—A positive monophasic action current. Membrane B is cooled to 1° C. Membrane A is stimulated. Depolarization of membrane A is rapid, as indicated by the steep upstroke; repolarization takes place more slowly, as indicated by the slowly declining downstroke in the tracing.

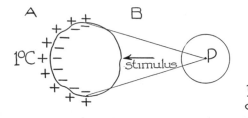
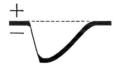

Resultant tracing is that of a negative monophasic action current

FIG. 31.—A negative monophasic action current.

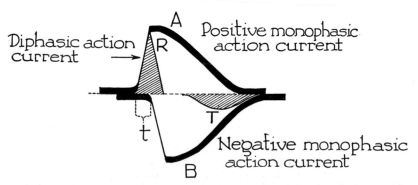

FIG. 32.—A diphasic action current (shaded) produced by the algebraic addition of the *positive monophasic action current* shown in figure 30 and the *negative monophasic action current* shown in figure 31.

Obviously, when membranes B and A are alternately cooled to 1° C. and the warm membrane depolarized and repolarized, the net result should be similar to that obtained and illustrated by figures 30 and 31 when each membrane is depolarized and repolarized in immediate succession. That the net result is really similar can be seen from figure 32, in which the two tracings of the monophasic action currents from each membrane are superimposed, the one produced by membrane A being made to begin slightly earlier than the one produced by membrane B. The interval in time (t, Fig. 32) between the onsets of the two tracings is equal to the time required for the depolarization wave of membrane A,

DEPOLARIZATION PROCESS

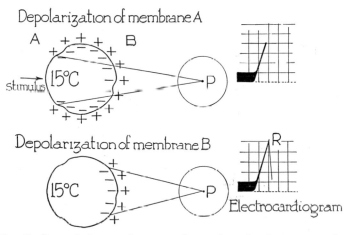

Fig. 33.—Cooling of the membrane produces slow *depolarization* and a slowly rising positive deflection of the string. When membrane B is reached, depolarization takes place at the more rapid normal rate and the downward deflection of the string is rapid.

started by a stimulus indicated by the arrow (Fig. 27), to reach around to membrane B. Therefore, from figure 32 and figure 27 it is seen that the tracing of a *diphasic action current is the algebraic sum of two monophasic action currents.*

If, instead of membrane A being cooled to 1° C., it is cooled to 15° C., the physicochemical processes will not be inhibited completely, but they will only be slowed. After membrane A is cooled to 15° C., it is stimulated at the point indicated by the arrow (Fig. 33). This produces deceleration of the depolarization process in that membrane and therefore results in an upstroke of the depolarization wave, which rises slowly and is *slurred* (see p. 83). When the impulse or depolarization process reaches membrane B, it moves rapidly again and thereby results in a sharp sudden decline of the downstroke of the depolarization wave (Fig. 33). Because membrane *A* is cool and the chemical processes are slowed, a much longer time is required for that membrane to reach the state of repolarization. Along the surface of the warmer membrane *B*, the chemical processes take place at a more rapid rate and therefore repolarization begins on its surface first. This results in a *positive deflection* of the galvanometer during repolarization or a *positive* repolarization wave (Fig. 34). Such shifts in direction of T waves resemble the T (repolarization) wave changes in the clinical electrocardiogram of man encountered in many physiologic and disease states.

REPOLARIZATION PROCESS

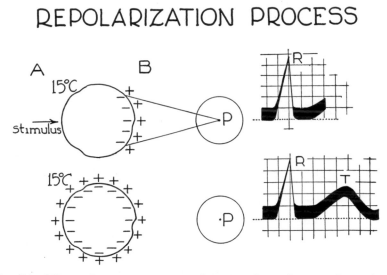

Fɪɢ. 34.—The repolarization wave is made positive by cooling membrane A to 15° C. and stimulating membrane A.

EFFECT OF POTASSIUM

When potassium, such as KCl, is added in the proper amounts to the surface of a polarized membrane, depolarization of the membrane occurs. The degree of depolarization varies directly with the amount of potassium ions applied. If KCl is applied to membrane *A* so as partially to depolarize it, the base line or isoelectric line is immediately shifted from zero potential to a positive or negative potential (Fig. 35). In figure 35 the shift takes place in a positive or upward direction because the point *P* is now in a field of relative positivity. This difference in potential is called the *current of injury*. It may also be brought about by other types of chemical injury and by physical injury, as by pinching the end of a strip of muscle or by reducing its oxygen supply locally.

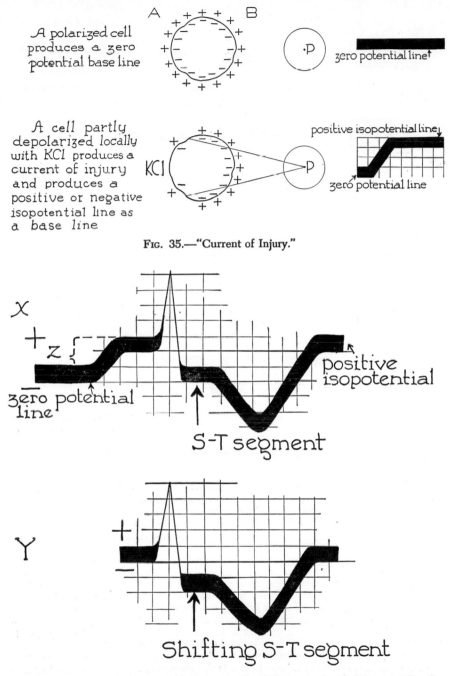

A polarized cell produces a zero potential base line

A cell partly depolarized locally with KCl produces a current of injury and produces a positive or negative isopotential line as a base line

zero potential line

positive isopotential line

zero potential line

Fig. 35.—"Current of Injury."

zero potential line

positive isopotential

S-T segment

Shifting S-T segment

Fig. 36.—When membrane A of the injured cell shown in figure 35 is stimulated, the tracing X results. On the finished electrocardiogram the shift Z is usually not seen and therefore the finished tracing has the appearance of tracing Y.

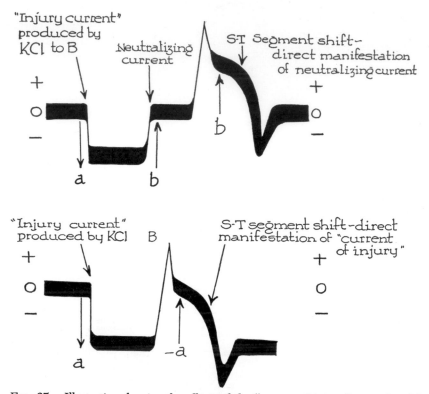

FIG. 37.—Illustration showing the effects of the "current of injury," *a*, produced by applying KCl to membrane B (Fig. 35), upon the S–T segment with and without the influence of a compensating or neutralizing current, *b*, from the control circuit of the electrocardiograph. Although the final configuration of the S–T segment in relation to the depolarization and repolarization complexes remain the same, the relationship of the S–T segment shift to the zero or isopotential line is altered by the compensating current. The S–T segment is shifted in a positive direction when KCl is applied to membrane B and in a negative direction (Fig. 36) when applied to membrane A, and the exploring electrode is opposite membrane B.

In the upper trace the addition of KCl to membrane B of the hypothetic cell resulted in partial depolarization of that membrane, thus creating a field of negative potential at the exploring electrode P. The string, therefore, deflects downward or in the negative direction by an electric force, *a*, representing the difference in potential between P and p. When the string is centered for recording, a compensating current is applied to the circuit of the string from the control box. This current, *b*, neutralizes the injury current *a*. When the cell is completely depolarized after a stimulus is applied (only partially if cell is not killed), the force *a*, due to the current of injury, is lost. This leaves the compensating current, *b*, unbalanced during the period of the excited state or when the S–T segment is inscribed. Therefore, the S–T segment is deflected in a positive direction because of the unbalanced *b* electric force.

The lower part of the figure shows the electric reactions when a compensating current is not employed in the recording; *a* is the current of injury due to the KCl and — *a* is the loss of this current during the depolarized or excited state.

If membrane *A* is now stimulated (Fig. 35) and the cell is depolarized and repolarized, the resultant tracing of these processes is as shown in figure 36. It is noted that the zero potential line, S–T segment (Fig. 36) between the depolarization and repolarization waves is "shifted" downward in relation to the positive isopotential line shown just before the depolarization wave and after the repolarization wave.

If potassium is applied to membrane *B* instead of *A*, the resultant current of injury will produce a negative shift in the isopotential line and a positive shift of the S–T segment instead of a negative one as shown in figure 36, *X* and *Y*.

When an electrocardiogram is taken, the shift in the isopotential line from one of zero potential to a positive or negative potential produced by a current of injury is not seen. The only evidence of the activity of a current of injury is a positive or negative deflection of the S–T segment. This is explained by the fact that the shadow of the string of the galvanometer is brought to the center of the camera by neutralizing all steady currents from the patient by means of a battery and resistors in the "control box." Among the currents so neutralized is the current of injury when it is present. For instance, if a current of injury produces a shift of the string to the negative side by one unit, then one positive unit of EMF is made to flow in the opposite direction. The string then moves to the zero position or center of the camera or the zero potential position. Now, when the muscle is depolarized, this extra positive unit of EMF from the control box is unbalanced and thereby results in a positive shift of the base line or isoelectric line during the depolarized state of the muscle (Fig. 37).

EFFECTS OF DEPOLARIZATION AND REPOLARIZATION OF THE HYPOTHETIC CELL UPON THE THREE STANDARD LEADS

The purpose of the foregoing discussion is to point out that by means of the galvanometer recordings it is possible to determine the *magnitude, i.e.,* the degree of EMF, the *sense, i.e.,* the positive or negative character, and the *direction* of the depolarization and repolarization processes in a living cell. By use of three galvanometers to record the three leads simultaneously, or by use of one galvanometer to record each lead alternately, as is usually done in taking the three standard leads, the *magnitude, sense,* and the *direction* of the depolarization or repolarization processes can be determined in the frontal plane for any time. Likewise, it is possible to visualize the behavior of the electric axis of the depolarization and repolarization processes from the finished tracings in the three limb leads.

In order to illustrate the foregoing points, the following arguments are presented: If the "cell," which is comparable to the human heart, is placed in a volume conductor and electrodes are led off in the manner indicated by figure 38, there results an electric situation which is analo-

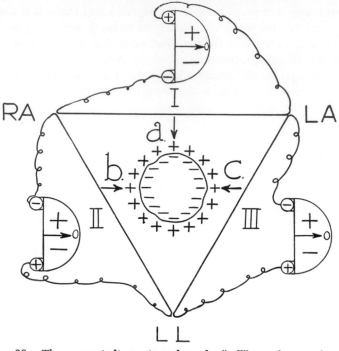

FIG. 38.—The arrows indicate sites where the "cell" is to be stimulated. (See text for explanation.)

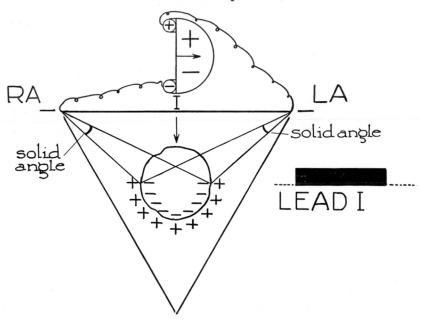

FIG. 39.—The depolarization process halfway around the cell and analyzed for lead I. The stimulus was applied at the top of the cell.

gous to that seen in man when the three standard leads are taken. It can be seen from figure 38 that the *RA, LA* and *LL* electrode connections form the apices of what is essentially an equilateral triangle. This is known as the *Einthoven triangle*.

Example I.—If the cell is stimulated at the point indicated by the arrow *a* in figure 38, the depolarization process travels from above downward.

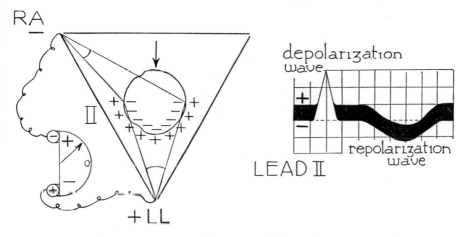

FIG. 40.—Depolarization process halfway around the cell and analyzed for lead II. The stimulus was applied at the top of the cell.

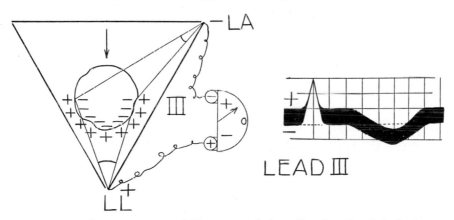

FIG. 41.—Depolarization process halfway around the cell and analyzed for lead III. The stimulus was applied at the top of the cell.

The solid angles at the *RA* and *LA* electrodes are equal and the electric fields are both negative as the observer standing at the *RA* and *LA* electrodes observes the negative charges during the depolarization process. Thus, there is no potential difference between the electrodes at *RA* and *LA*, and therefore no current flows during depolarization or repolarization of the cell. No deflections of the string are seen in lead I (Fig. 39).

In lead II the solid angle at the *LL* electrode is large and the electric field is positive (Fig. 40). At *RA* electrode the angle is small and the field is negative. Whenever the *RA* is relatively negative and the *LL* relatively positive in lead II, an upright or positive deflection is written. Since repolarization starts where depolarization began, an inverted repolarization wave is written in lead II (Fig. 40).

Lead III, which is shown in figure 41, is identical with lead II for the same reasons.

The three standard leads then appear as shown in figure 42 when the stimulus is applied to the upper part of the cell.

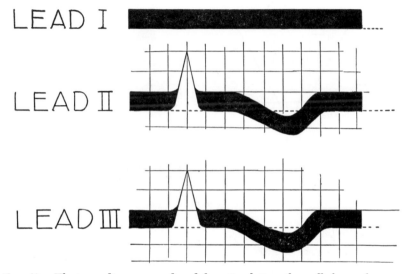

Fɪɢ. 42.—Electrocardiogram produced by stimulating the cell from above, as indicated by arrow (*a*) in figure 38.

Example II.—If the membrane is stimulated at the point indicated by arrow *b*, figure 38, and the depolarization process travels from right to left, there results a large upright deflection in lead I, since the solid angle is large and negative at the *RA* electrode and is equally large and positive at the *LA* electrode. The potential difference between these electrodes is large, and therefore a deflection of large amplitude is produced in lead I. Since the *RA* electrode is relatively negative and the *LA* electrode relatively positive, the deflection of the string is positive or upright. If the solid angle at *RA* represents a potential of — 2 units and the solid angle at the *LA* electrode represents a force of + 2 units, the potential difference between the two electrodes is 4 units and a deflection of the string of this magnitude is produced (Fig. 43). Repolarization produces a negative wave.

In the case of lead II the *RA* electrode is in a strong negative field and the *LL* electrode is in a field of zero potential (Fig. 44). If the force at the *RA* electrode is — 2 units and that at the *LL* electrode is 0 unit, the algebraic difference would be 2 units, which represents the force acting between the two electrodes. Thus, a deflection for lead II may be drawn with an amplitude of 2 units (Fig. 44). It is upright, since the *RA* electrode is negative and the *LL* electrode is positive. Repolarization produces a negative deflection.

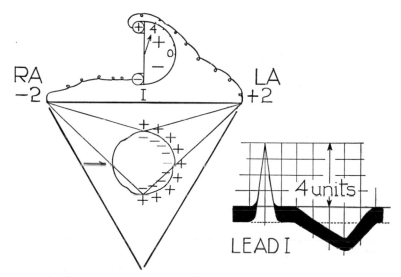

FIG. 43.—The depolarization process halfway around the cell and analyzed from the point of view of lead I. The stimulus was applied at the right of the "cell."

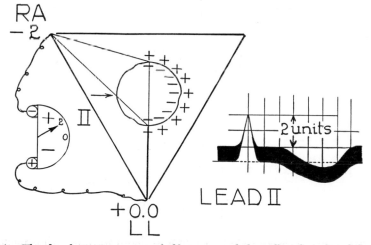

FIG. 44.—The depolarization process halfway around the cell and analyzed from the point of view of lead II. The stimulus was applied at the right of the cell.

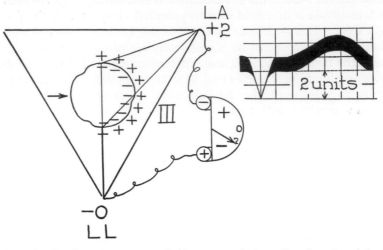

FIG. 45.—The depolarization process halfway around the cell and analyzed for lead III. The stimulus was applied at the right of the cell.

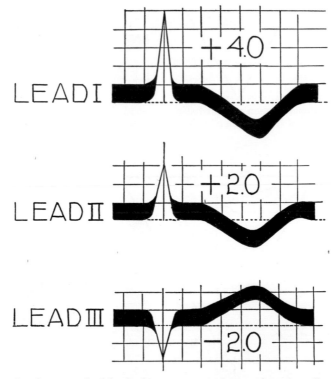

FIG. 46.—The three standard leads then appear as shown when the cell is stimulated at its right (arrow *b*, Fig. 38.).

In lead III the *LA* electrode is in a strongly positive field arbitrarily given as + 2 units; the *LL* electrode is in a zero potential field or 0 unit. The algebraic difference is 2 units. The direction of the deflection is *negative*, since the *LA* electrode is of relatively greater positivity than the *LL* electrode (Fig. 45). The deflection is down, or negative. It has been stated and shown previously that in order to standardize electrocardiography throughout the world, the connections between the subject and the galvanometer are so made that whenever the left arm electrode is rela-

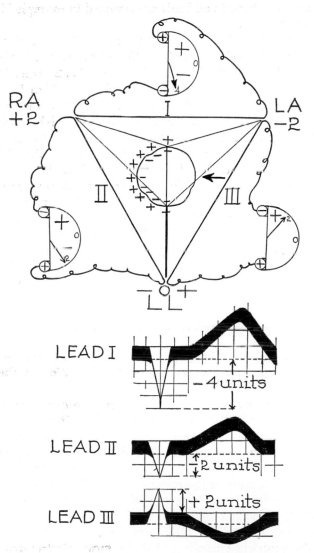

FIG. 47.—The effects of depolarization and repolarization on the electrodes and resultant tracings in the standard leads when the stimulus is applied at the left of of the cell (see *c*, Fig. 38).

4

tively negative and the left leg electrode is relatively positive, the galvanometer produces a *positive* deflection.

Example III.—If the cell is stimulated at the point indicated by arrow *c*, figure 38, and the depolarization process travels from left to right, the effects of depolarization and repolarization on the electrodes of the three standard leads and the resultant tracings are shown in figure 47. In this instance the polarity of the *RA* and *LA* is reversed when compared with that in example II, and therefore directions of the depolarization and repolarization deflections in all leads are reversed in example III as compared with example II.

The preceding discussions show that the mean direction of depolarization will influence the relative configuration of the waves in the finished tracings for the three standard leads. The reverse is also true. The waves in the tracings of the three standard leads, when considered collectively, indicate the mean direction of the depolarization process in the "cell" or in the human heart (see below, The Mean Electric Axis). It will be seen later that the electrocardiographic tracings illustrated in the preceding three examples suggest the pictures seen in patients with: (1) a ptotic heart, (2) left axis deviation, and (3) right axis deviation.

If the stimulus is applied directly posteriorly or anteriorly or within the center of the homogeneous cell, so that the depolarization process spreads uniformly from the point of stimulation, no depolarization or repolarization waves are seen in the standard leads, since no differences in potential between the electrodes result. The precordial leads to be discussed later are employed to detect electric currents flowing perpendicularly to the frontal plane. These should be recorded routinely in clinical electrocardiography.

THE MEAN ELECTRIC AXIS

It is advisable to determine routinely the magnitude and direction of the mean electric axis of the process of depolarization in the finished human electrocardiogram.

The mean electric axis may be described for the depolarization or repolarization processes of the auricles or ventricles. It may be defined as the mean electromotive force (magnitude) of depolarization or repolarization, acting in an average direction during the period of electric activity. It is a *vector quantity* in that it has *magnitude, direction* and *sense.* It may be defined as the mean electric axis of the depolarization process of the auricle (usually termed the *mean electric axis of the P wave*), or of the depolarization process of the ventricle (usually termed the *mean electric axis of the QRS complex*), or of the repolarization process of the ventricle (usually called the *mean electric axis of the T wave*). We have seen the mean electric axes derived for the hypothetic "cell."

The axis may best be represented by a *vector force* (Fig. 48), the length of which represents the magnitude or quantity of the current. The spatial direction is represented by the position of the vector, with the head of the arrow indicating the direction of action of the current or electric force. The polarity or sense of the vector is such that the head is relatively positive and the tail relatively negative. Current flows in the direction indicated by the vector and always travels from the negative to the positive end.

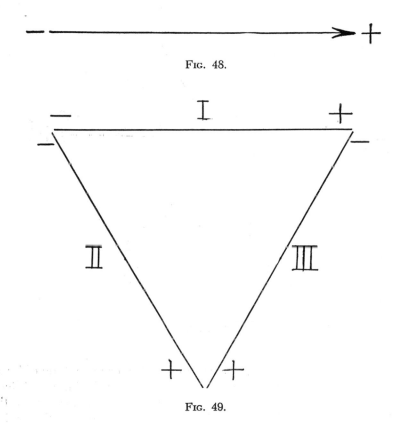

FIG. 48.

FIG. 49.

The mean electric axis may be determined by numerous methods, three of which will be presented.

I. The Triaxial Reference System.—The triaxial reference system, as described by R. H. Bayley, may be used as a simple means of determining the mean electric axis of any wave of depolarization or repolarization from the electrocardiogram. Based upon Einthoven's triangle, it is constructed as follows: If a point is placed midway between the ends of each limb lead line in the Einthoven triangle (Fig. 49) and each limb lead line of the triangle is transposed in space so that the points are superimposed, an axial system will thus be formed (Fig. 50). The limbs form 60° angles with each other. The axial system is divided into degrees or parts of two hemicircles, so that the direction of the electric axis may be defined. The three o'clock axis is labeled 0 degree, and directional measurements are made from it. The other angles are labeled about the zero degree axis as shown in figure 50.

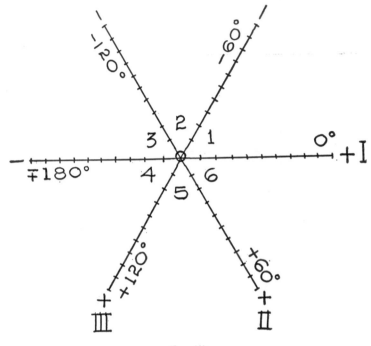

Fɪɢ. 50.

In order to measure the electric axes in quantity or magnitude of force, the axial system is arbitrarily divided into units along the limb lead lines. That portion of the lead I line from the center of the axial system to the terminus at the 0° point is +, the other half is —; that part of the lead II line from the center or zero point of the axial system to the terminus at the + 60° point is +, the other half is —; and that part of the lead III line from the center of the axial system to the terminus at the + 120° point is +, the other half is —; (Fig. 50). Consult the Appendix, figure 285 for minute details of the triaxial reference system and become thoroughly acquainted with it to the point of being able to draw one accurately by free hand and in detail. This will be of considerable use in the electric analysis of electrocardiograms from the point of view of the ventricular gradient as well as of the mean electric axis. It is a powerful tool in electrocardiography.

Analysis of the mean electric axis of any complex, with the use of the triaxial system, is made from any two of the three standard leads recorded with the galvanometer properly standardized. It is customary to use leads I and III. The algebraic sum in millimeters of the amplitudes of the positive waves and of the negative waves in lead I is plotted on the lead I axis. The algebraic sum of the amplitudes of the positive waves and

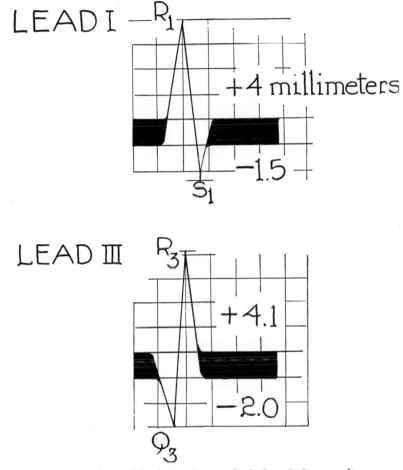

FIG. 51.—Lead I and lead III of a standard clinical electrocardiogram.

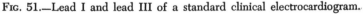

of the negative waves in lead III is plotted on the lead III axis. Perpendicular lines are dropped through the point plotted on the lead lines. The mean electric axis is a vector force represented by a line drawn from the center of the triaxial reference system to the point of intersection of the perpendiculars, the head of the arrow being placed at this point of intersection. The length of the vector in units, equal to those represented on the lead lines, represents the mean EMF; the number of degrees the vector force makes with the zero line represents its mean direction; and the sign + or − represents its sense, the + sign at the head of the arrow representing the vector.

It is well to point out at this time that a vector (manifest vector) so derived represents a spatial vector projected upon the frontal plane, *i.e.*, a plane with its surface parallel to the anterior surface of the body. A discussion of spatial, scalar, and vector quantities will not be entered into here.

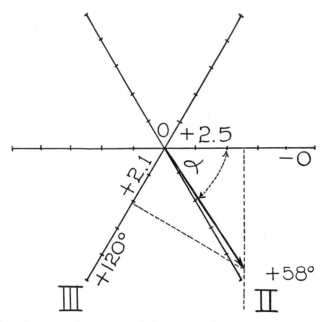

Fig. 52.—The mean electric axis of the tracing shown in figure 51 as plotted on the triaxial reference system.

Example.—The mean electric axis for the QRS is determined as follows: In figure 51, R_1 measures + 4 millimeters and S_1 measures − 1.5 millimeters, a difference of +2.5 millimeters. This is plotted on the positive side of the lead I line as 2.5 arbitrary units (Fig. 52). R_3 measures + 4.1 and Q_3 −2.0 millimeters; the difference is +2.1 millimeters. This is marked off on the lead III line on the positive side. Perpendiculars to leads I and III are drawn through the plotted points. The mean electric axis is drawn from the 0 point or center of the triaxial reference system to the point of intersection of the perpendiculars and is indicated by the arrow, with the head at the point of the intersection. It is a true *vector force.*

In this example the magnitude of the mean electric axis is approximately 5 units, the direction is +58°, as indicated by the angle α. Practice this procedure of analysis until the method is mastered.

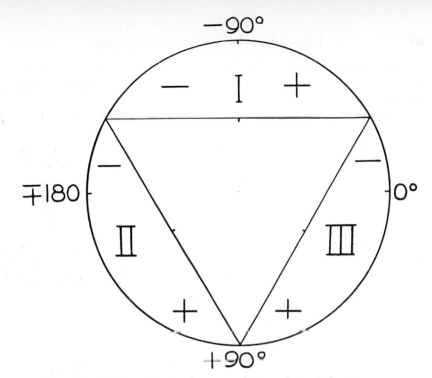

FIG. 53.—Einthoven's triangle arranged for analysis of electric axes.

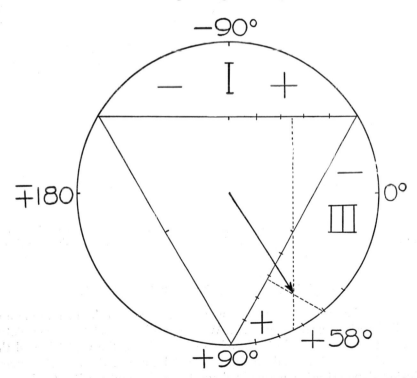

FIG. 54.—The mean electric axis of the QRS plotted on the Einthoven's triangle.

(55)

II. Dieuaide's Chart.—This is shown in the Appendix, figure 286, and may be used to determine the mean electric axis. Its method of use is also described in the Appendix.

III. Einthoven's Triangle.—Arrange Einthoven's triangle as shown in figure 53.

Example.—The mean electric axis of QRS is determined as follows: The algebraic sum of R_1 and S_1 (+2.5 mm.) is plotted on the lead I line. (The values used in this example are the same as those in figure 51.) A perpendicular to lead I is drawn through this point. The difference between R_3 and Q_3 is +2.1 millimeters. This is plotted on the positive portion of the lead III line, and a line is drawn through this point perpendicular to the lead III line. The mean electric axis is represented by a line drawn from the center of the triangle to the point of intersection of the perpendiculars (Fig. 54). The values of the resultant vector are the same as in the previous one (Fig. 52).

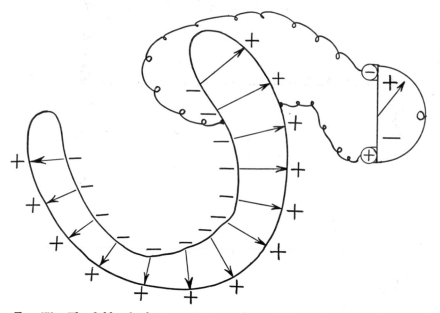

Fig. 55.—The fields of relative positivity and negativity in the ventricular muscle during depolarization. The arrows and the + and − signs indicate the direction of migration of the depolarization process.

THE HEART AS A POLARIZED "CELL"

The cardiac muscle acts in a manner analogous to the membrane and "cell" described previously. F. N. Wilson and his associates have pointed out that if one electrode is placed in the cavity of the ventricle and the other electrode is placed on the epicardial surface, the electric current during depolarization normally flows from the endocardial to the epicardial surface of the heart. As the depolarization impulse travels through the myocardium, a positive charge (the source) precedes and a negative charge (the sink) follows the wave of depolarization. Thus, the electrode inside the ventricle is relatively negative and the electrode on the surface of the ventricle is relatively positive (Fig. 55).

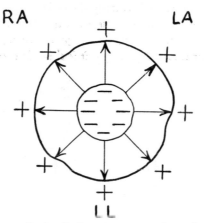

FIG. 56.—Forces acting equally in all directions in a spherical mass of muscle would result in no EMF in the standard limb leads.

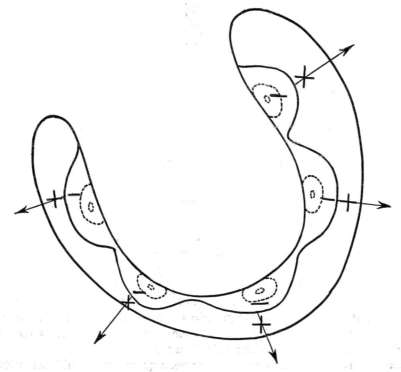

FIG. 57.—The form of the ventricles may be considered as an irregularly shaped U. The dotted lines indicate the previous positions of the depolarization wave at an earlier instant.

If the heart were a completely enclosed sphere of muscle and the electric forces acted equally in all directions, no potential difference would be detected by the ordinary electrodes employed clinically and no electrocardiogram or potential differences would be recorded (Fig. 56). The ventricles, however, are not a completely enclosed sphere of muscle. In fact, they form a more or less irregularly U shaped shell with the open portion at the base in the region of the artrioventricular valves. *It is because of this open region, in large measure, that electric forces detectable by the ordinary types of clinical leads result* (Fig. 57).

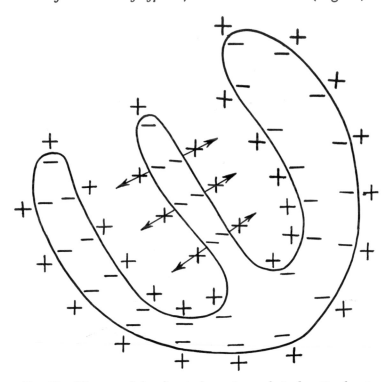

FIG. 58.—Diagram of the electric forces in a polarized resting heart.

The interventricular septum, with its more or less equal and opposite forces, normally exerts its influence on the electrodes to a negligible extent, depending in large part upon the position of the electrodes in relation to the heart (Fig. 58). The septal Q originates in the septum.

It is advisable to point out here that the electric axis is continually changing in direction and magnitude as depolarization of the cardiac musculature progresses. It is not a single static vector force, as the discussion immediately preceding might suggest.

The electric axis of the ventricles has been given considerable attention, whereas that of the auricles has not. In fact, only the depolarization complex of the ventricles (QRS) has, therefore, received much attention, and only recently has the repolarization process of the ventricle, represented by the T wave, received study.

The direction of the axis is dependent upon many factors, such as the health of the muscle and the relative thicknesses and positions of the ventricular walls. If the electric axis is plotted at *any given instant* during the depolarization process, there is derived a vector force which is termed the *mean instantaneous electric axis*. The average direction and

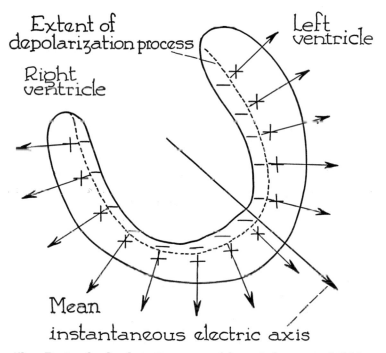

FIG. 59.— During the depolarization process (shown to have extended 30 per cent of the way through the ventricular muscular mass) many doublets are formed which, when added as vector quantities, constitute the *mean instantaneous electric axis* at that particular moment in the depolarization process. Each doublet produces a force, represented by the arrows, running from the negative to the positive pole.

magnitude of all of the *mean* instantaneous electric axes produced during depolarization of the ventricles constitute the *mean electric axis of the QRS complex*, or the mean electric axis for the entire depolarization process. The average directions and magnitudes of all of the *mean* instantaneous electric axes during depolarization of the auricles constitute the *mean electric axis of the P wave*. The same definitions hold for the repolarization processes. These may be applied for the entire heart as a unit or for any part separately.

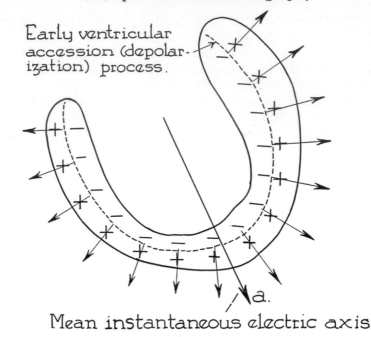

Early ventricular accession (depolarization) process.

Mean instantaneous electric axis

Fig. 60.—The mean instantaneous electric axis at the *beginning of depolarization* of the ventricular musculature.

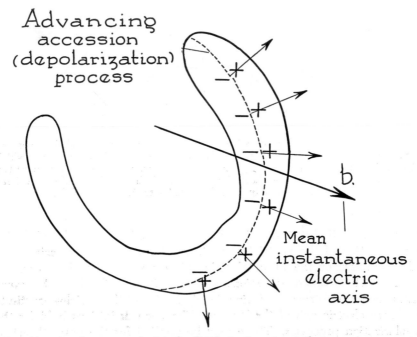

Advancing accession (depolarization) process

Mean instantaneous electric axis

Fig. 61.—*At a later stage during the depolarization process* the mean instantaneous axis points more to the left (a counterclockwise movement of the axis) than during the early stage of depolarization shown in figure 60.

The Instantaneous Electric Axis.—The *mean instantaneous electric axis and the mean electric axis of the QRS complex are shown in figures 59 through 63.* The wall of the right ventricle is thin, whereas that of the left ventricle is relatively thick. Stimuli starting in the Purkinje system at numerous points on the endocardial surface of the myocardium spread more or less equally and perpendicular to the epicardial surface. The sum of these forces at any instant is the *mean instantaneous electric axis* for the whole heart at a period during a particular depolarization process (Fig. 59).

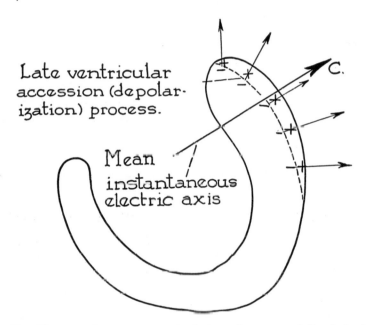

Late ventricular accession (depolar-ization) process.

Mean instantaneous electric axis

C.

FIG. 62.—The mean instantaneous axis during a *late* stage of depolarization.

The vector sum of the mean instantaneous electric axes is equal to the mean QRS axis.

In figure 60, the average direction of the electric forces during *early depolarization* is from the base to the apex of the ventricles, as there are no forces present at the base of the heart to counteract those acting at the apex. The forces on the sides of the ventricles are essentially equal and opposite and tend to neutralize each other.

A *few moments later, as the depolarization wave progresses,* it has passed through the relatively thin right ventricle but is still traveling through the thick wall of the left ventricle. At this later instant the *mean* instantaneous axis has moved to the left (Fig. 61).

At an extremely *late stage during the depolarization process,* only a few doublets remain in the thicker regions of the left ventricle. These forces produce a mean instantaneous axis which is rotated still farther to the left (Fig. 62).

Thus, it may be seen that the mean instantaneous electric axis may be indicated by a vector drawn from the center of the ventricles to the average direction of the forces produced by the doublets. If the mean instantaneous axes shown in figures 60, 61, and 62 are added vectorially, the *mean electric axis of the QRS complex* is obtained (Fig. 63).

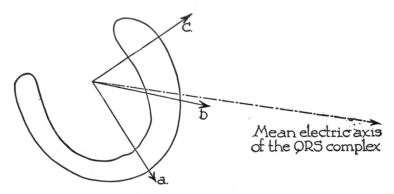

FIG. 63.—By addition of the instantaneous electric axes *a*, *b*, and *c*, the *mean electric axis of the QRS complex* is obtained.

THE MONOCARDIOGRAM OR VECTORCARDIOGRAM

In ordinary analysis of the electric axis for clinical purposes, the mean electric axis of the QRS complex is the only one studied. It is possible, however, if any two of the three standard leads are recorded simultaneously to determine the electric axis of any of the waves or complexes at any one instant during the depolarization or repolarization process of the atrial or ventricular musculature. There is, mathematically speaking, an almost unlimited number of such axes that may be determined for each wave or complex. (The QRS complex has been the one studied most.) All that is usually done, however, is to measure several mean instantaneous axes for consecutive periods during the depolarization complex and record them as indicated in the following example. The resultant of these axes can be expressed as a *loop*, commonly spoken of as the *QRS loop*, or the *Monocardiogram* of Mann or the *Vectorcardiogram* of Wilson and his associates. With the use of the cathode ray oscillograph the entire analysis can be made electrically, the loop alone being recorded. Although it is beyond the purpose of this presentation to discuss the circuit of this recorder, it is felt that the *monocardiogram* is sufficiently important to warrant a discussion of the method used by Mann to convert tracings recorded by ordinary standard leads into the picture of the changing electric axis or the vectorcardiogram. Another method is shown in figure 251 of Chapter 5.

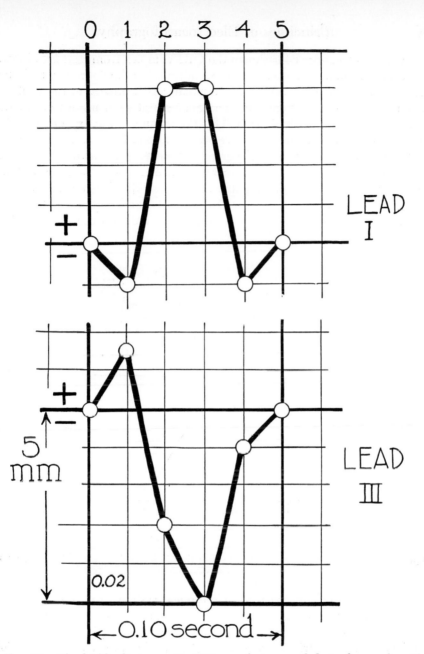

Fig. 64.—The highly diagrammatic QRS complexes recorded simultaneously with properly standardized galvanometers for leads I and III, from which the monocardiogram or vectorcardiogram was constructed for the accompanying discussions. The isoelectric lines are shown between the + and − signs. Positive deflections are above and negative deflections are below these lines. The time lines occur every 0.02 second, indicated by the lines labeled 0, 1, 2, 3, 4, 5. Analyses of the mean instantaneous electric axes of the QRS complex are found at these time intervals. The amplitude is measured in millimeters. The circles on the waves represent points at which the mean instantaneous electric axes are determined. For this illustration the camera was made to move more rapidly than is customary in order to spread the complex over a greater area and facilitate the analysis.

Example.—In figure 64 is shown the QRS complex from lead I and lead III recorded simultaneously. Points are indicated in the figure at which the electric axis of the QRS complex or depolarization process of the ventricular musculature is determined. The analyses at each instant are made in the manner previously described for the mean electric axis of the QRS complex (see p. 50). The *triaxial reference system* is used. For example, at the moment during the depolarization process indicated by point 1, figure 64, the Q wave is —1 millimeter in lead I, and at the same instant (found by referring to the vertical time lines) the R wave in lead III measures +1.5 millimeters. The —1 is located 1 unit on the negative side of the lead I line and the +1.5 is located 1.5 units on the positive side

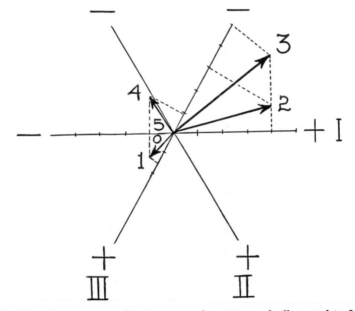

Fig. 65.—Mean instantaneous electric axes at the six intervals illustrated in figure 64.

of the lead III line of the triaxial reference system (Fig. 65). Perpendicular lines are drawn to each of these lead lines through the points found. The point of intersection of the perpendicular lines is connected to the center of the triaxial system with the head of the arrow at the point of intersection of the perpendicular lines. The resultant is a *vector* force representing the force of the depolarization process as projected upon the frontal plane at 0.02 second from its onset. The same analysis was repeated at 0.02 second intervals in this example from the time of onset to the completion of the depolarization of the ventricular musculature. This results in many vector forces that occur in sequence. In this example there are six such forces, the first and last ones being zero. These *mean instantaneous vector forces* are transposed from the triaxial system, as shown in figure 66. The tips of the arrows are connected serially by a dotted line, which moves in a counterclockwise direction. This resultant *QRS loop* is called the *monocardiogram* or *vectorcardiogram* and indicates vectorially in rather detailed fashion the magnitude and direction of the

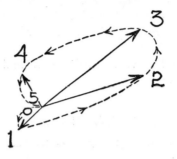

FIG. 66.—The monocardiogram or vectorcardiogram derived from the QRS complexes shown in figure 64.

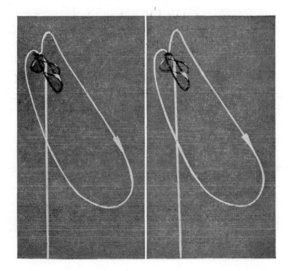

FIG. 67.—P, QRS, and T sE-loops of a normal individual. This figure may be viewed stereoscopically by placing a card between the two portions of the illustration and slowly moving the illustration away or toward one's eyes until a three-dimensional relationship is observed.

depolarization process in the ventricular musculature during various stages of that one particular depolarization process.

Mann's method of analysis is tedious. As previously mentioned, the cathode ray oscillograph can be used but its expense and the state of the present information concerning the QRS loop make it generally impractical. Nevertheless, since its use may at some future date become general, an understanding of the vectorcardiogram is warranted. Furthermore, it gives insight into the dynamic and unstable nature of the depolarization and repolarization processes, justifying at least a knowledge of the vector-cardiogram.

Future developments in electrocardiography necessitate an evaluation of the spatial relationship of the electric phenomena associated with cardiac activity. A normal spatial vectorcardiogram is illustrated in Figure 67.

The method of recording vectorcardiograms and their significance are discussed briefly on page 249.

EINTHOVEN'S LAW

One of Kirchoff's laws states that the algebraic sum of all electric forces flowing to a single point in a network is equal to zero. *Einthoven's law* states that the algebraic sum of any complex in lead I and the complex in lead III recorded at the same instant is equal to the complex recorded in lead II at that instant. From the previous discussions, it is obvious that such a law applies to electrocardiography and that *Einthoven's law* is true. This is readily seen when the three standard leads are recorded simultaneously. This law has many practical and theoretic applications. Incidentally, it is useful for checking errors in mounting and labeling electrocardiograms. This law may be applied even if each lead is recorded separately, but, of course, the necessary allowances must be made for respiration and changes in mechanism which occur between the recording of any two leads.

Chapter 2

AN ANALYSIS OF VARIOUS COMPONENTS OF THE ELECTROCARDIOGRAM AND THEIR CLINICAL SIGNIFICANCE

In the discussions to follow, concerning the components of the electrocardiogram, it is necessary that the reader visualize the depolarization and repolarization processes, currents of injury, and other electric phenomena presented in the previous chapter. To memorize certain facts without understanding the accepted explanations of the mechanisms involved in the electric activity leads to failure of purpose and reduces the study of electrocardiography to a course in memorizing patterns. The student loses interest in the problem of electrocardiography and is ultimately so discouraged that no further applications of effort are made. Only with a thorough understanding of the accepted mechanisms involved is it possible to gain some insight into the applications and limitations of electrocardiography in various cardiac states in health and disease.

ARTIFACTS

Before interpretation of an electrocardiogram is attempted, it is necessary to make certain that no technical difficulties have made the tracing

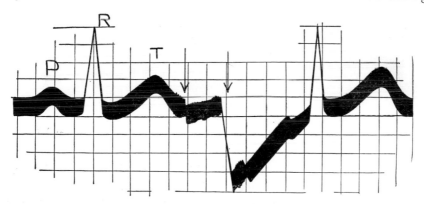

Fig. 68.—Artifacts due to movement of the subject. The artifacts are indicated by the arrows. The fine fibrillary vibrations in the isoelectric line are due to muscular contractions, the sudden large movements to slipping of the electrodes over the skin at the point of contact. It is noted that they show no basic rhythm, occur suddenly, vary considerably and are superimposed upon the components of the electrocardiogram. The artifacts usually can be identified even though the tracing is often extremely distorted.

unfit for interpretation. Among these are certain *artifacts* which are seldom confusing. The more common ones include:

1. *Movement of the Patient.*—Movement on the part of the patient with associated contraction of the skeletal muscles results in sudden changes in current conducted through the galvanometer, which produce sudden deflections (Figs. 68 and 72). In addition, movement of the subject disturbs the contacts of the electrodes on the body, which in turn causes

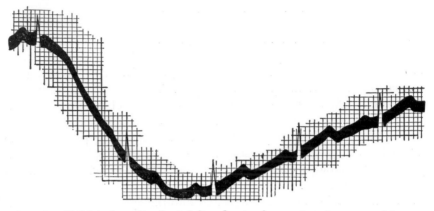

Fig. 69.—Shiftinig base (isoelectic) line due to changes in cutaneous resistance.

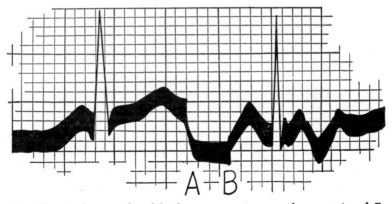

Fig. 70.—Artifacts produced by loose connections are shown at *A* and *B*.

changes in the resistance between the skin and the electrodes and results in movement of the galvanometer string (Fig. 68).

2. *Shifting in the base (isoelectric) line* is often due to cutaneous currents, polarization of electrodes, variations in cutaneous resistance, or swinging of wires conducting electricity close to the leads inducing current in the respective leads (Fig. 69).

3. *Loose contacts any place in the circuit* produce sudden shifting of the base line (Fig. 70).

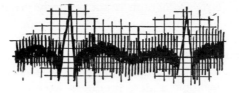

FIG. 71.—Artifacts due to interference by alternating 60 cycle current.

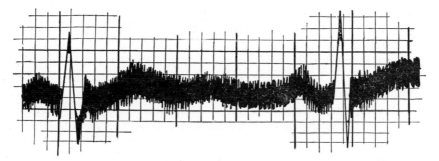

FIG. 72.—Artifacts due to muscular tremor.

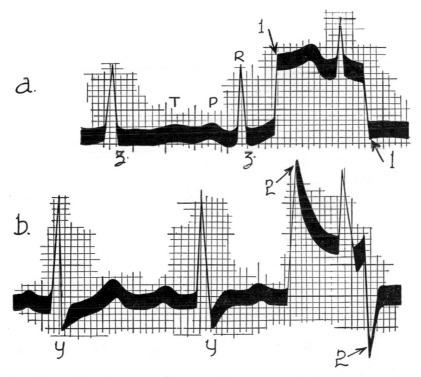

FIG. 73.—*a*, Normal electrocardiogram with proper standardization and tension on the string. *b*, Artifacts due to overshooting, producing definite slurring of the S wave and widening of the QRS complex, *Y*. No overshooting is present in the standardization at arrows (*1*), although it is seen at arrows (*2*).

4. When the electrocardiograph is not properly grounded or shielded, *alternating current* may produce regular fibrillary deflections at a rate of 60 times a second in 60 cycle alternating current. Notching or slurring of the complexes may also be produced (Fig. 71).

5. *Muscular tremor* of the skeletal muscles, such as is seen especially in psychogenic or neurologic states, produces irregular vibrations in the base line (Fig. 72). These vibrations differ from those due to alternating currents, which are regular in rate and uniform in height.

6. *Overshooting* may be produced by a loose string. The movement of such a string does not stop abruptly when a millivolt is added to or removed from the galvanometer circuit (Fig. 73, *b, 2*). When the string has a proper tension, the isoelectric line stops abruptly after being shifted by the change of 1 millivolt in the galvanometer circuit (Fig. 73, *a, 1*). Overshooting results in an abnormally high amplitude of the deflections with slurring and widening of the complexes, especially of those associated with extreme changes in the EMF (Fig. 73, *b, Y*). Each lead should be so standardized that when 1 millivolt of potential difference is introduced, a deflection of only 10 millimeters will be produced in the electrocardiogram with no overshooting (Fig. 73, *a, Z*).

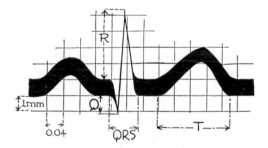

Fig. 74.—The duration of the QRS complex in this example is measured from the beginning of the convex surface of the Q wave to the end of the convex surface of the R wave. Measurements for the other waves, such as the P or T, are made in the same manner. The amplitude of the R wave is measured from the superior portion of the isoelectric line to the top of the wave. The Q wave is measured from the inferior portion of the isoelectric line to the apex of the wave.

METHODS FOR OBTAINING THE MEASUREMENTS

It is customary to measure the duration of the complexes, intervals and segments from their *convex curvatures* and not from their concave curvatures (Fig. 74) and to express the amplitude in millimeters or millivolts. The amplitude of the positive deflections may be conveniently measured from the superior portion of the isoelectric line to the apex of the wave in question, and the negative deflections may be measured from the inferior portion of the isoelectric line to the apex of the wave in question. This automatically corrects for the width of the string (Fig. 74).

Measurement of the ventricular rate is made in the following manner. A QRS complex that falls on or close to a heavy time line is selected. Fifteen heavy time lines are counted from it, and the number of QRS complexes falling within this unit of time (3.0 sec.) is counted. The interval of time between each complex represents a cycle of the ventricle, and fractions of time between two QRS complexes represent fractions of a cycle. Therefore, the number of QRS complexes times 20 is equal to the number of ventricular contractions falling within a 60 second period. The factor 20 is used for conversion to beats per minute. The auricular and ventricular rates should be counted separately, unless a P wave precedes each QRS complex, in which case the auricular rate is equal to the ventricular rate (Fig. 75). In practice, estimations of cardiac rate are

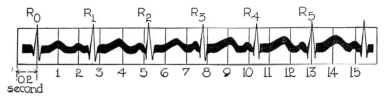

Fig. 75.—Determination of the cardiac rate. In the example, the number of R waves falling within 15 successive 0.20 second intervals is 5.9; 5.9 times 20 is 118, which is the ventricular rate per minute. Since a P wave precedes each R wave, the auricular rate is 118 per minute.

made at a glance from the length of the cardiac cycle. For example, if the interval in time between two successive R waves is 0.20 second or the interval of one heavy time line, the cardiac rate is 300 beats per minute; if the interval is 0.40 second or the interval of two heavy 0.20 second time lines, the rate is 150; if four heavy time lines, the rate is 75; five heavy 0.20 second time lines represent a rate of 60 and the like. It is easy to estimate the rate for fractions of 0.20 second heavy time line intervals. The rate is also equal to $\dfrac{60}{\text{R–R interval}}$.

THE P WAVE

The principal function of the SA node is to initiate at regular intervals impulses which act as stimuli for depolarization processes in the auricular and ventricular musculature. The depolarization process travels through the auricular musculature to the AV node. The impulses spread more or less equally in all directions from the SA node. The general course through the auricular wall is parallel with the endocardial and epicardial surfaces. The wave of depolarization spreads much as waves spread around the site where a pebble is dropped into a still pond of water. Preceding this depolarization wave, sometimes referred to as the *accession wave*, is the positive pole, the *source*, of a doublet and following it is the negative pole, the *sink* (Fig. 76). This depolarization process in the auricles is responsible for the differences in electric potential which result in the deflections inscribing the *P wave*.

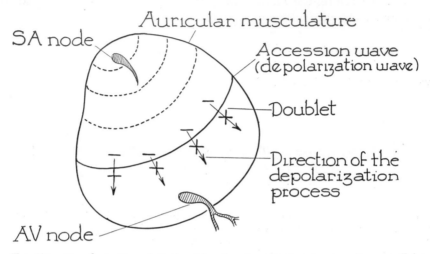

FIG. 76.—Depolarization of the auricles showing the impulse traveling parallel to the walls of the auricular muscle, with the *source* indicated by the + charge and the *sink* by the − charge. The dotted lines represent previous positions of the wave of depolarization.

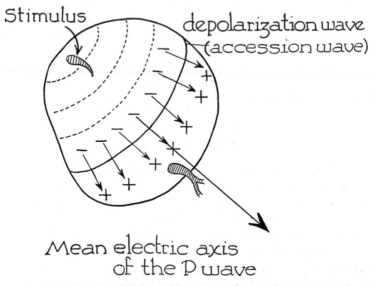

FIG. 77.—Depolarization of a sphere of auricular muscle.

The *wave of accession* or depolarization travels over the auricular muscle in three dimensions and may be depicted as passing over the surface of a *sphere* of muscle, the auricles (Fig. 77). The time-course or order of the depolarization process determines the direction and configuration of the depolarization wave of the auricle (P wave).

Figure 78 illustrates the manner in which the accession or depolarization wave in the auricles is responsible for differences in potential between the electrodes of the three standard leads. These differences in electric

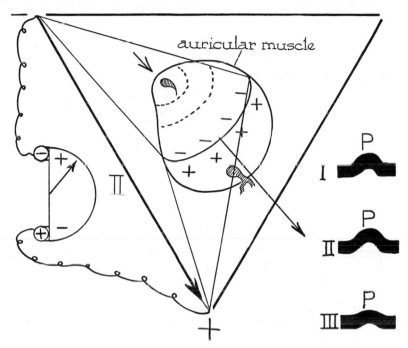

auricular muscle

P
I

P
II

P
III

FIG. 78.—A large P wave is written in lead II, as the mean electric axis of the P wave is essentially parallel to the lead II line.

potential are responsible for the EMF represented by the *P waves* in the three leads. It is easy to imagine how variations in the direction of the migration of the depolarization wave may produce variations in the configuration of the P wave, such as inversion, diphasicity, and the like.

The upper limits of normal for the P wave have been given in figure 5 and in the Appendix, Table 2. This wave is usually of greatest amplitude in lead II (Fig. 78). It is ordinarily *upright in leads I and II* but may be *upright, diphasic or inverted in lead III*, depending upon the average direction of travel of the auricular process of depolarization. Whenever the amplitude of the P wave exceeds 2.5 millimeters, it is considered *high*. When its duration is greater than 0.11 second, it is said to be *wide*. When the P wave is upright, it is said to be *positive;* when inverted, it is *nega-*

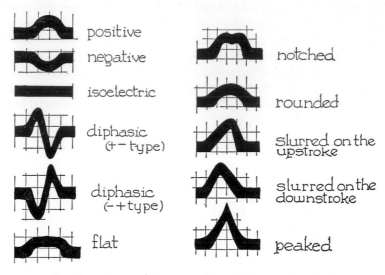

positive

negative

isoelectric

diphasic
(+ − type)

diphasic
(− + type)

flat

notched

rounded

slurred on the
upstroke

slurred on the
downstroke

peaked

Fig. 79.—Types of P waves. (See text for explanation.)

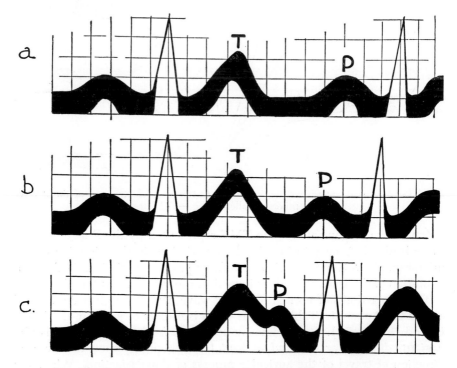

Fig. 80.—The P wave is sometimes difficult to identify when the cardiac rate is rapid. *a,* Relatively slow cardiac rate, T–P interval relatively long. *b,* More rapid rate, T–P interval short. *c,* Extremely rapid cardiac rate, the P wave is in the preceding T wave. Note that the T wave is deformed by the P wave.

tive. It may be *diphasic of the plus-minus type,* or *diphasic of the minus-plus type;* the latter is rarely found in the normal state. The wave may be *flat, round,* or *notched,* or it may be *slurred* along any part. Figure 79 illustrates variations in the configurations of the P wave. The presence of a P wave is definite evidence that the auricular musculature has been depolarized. The frequency, magnitude, duration, and direction of the depolarization process can be determined from the frequency, amplitude, duration, and positivity or negativity of the P waves in the standard leads of the electrocardiogram.

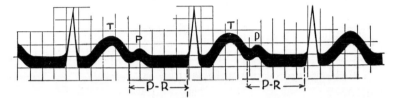

Fig. 81.—The P wave is superimposed upon the downstroke of the preceding T wave because of a prolongation of the P–R interval.

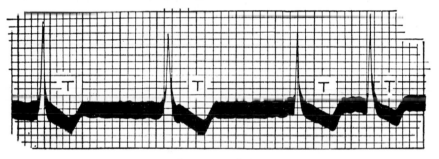

Fig. 82.—Auricular fibrillation. No definite P waves are present.

One of the practical problems in electrocardiography is identification of the P waves, which may be made difficult by a number of factors, among which are:

1. The P waves may be *isoelectric,* as in electrocardiograms showing low voltage, and are therefore difficult to identify. Fortunately, however, the P waves are usually prominent in at least one lead.

2. When the *cardiac rate increases,* the T–P interval shortens until the T and P waves become superimposed (Fig. 80). It may be difficult or even impossible to identify the P wave (Fig. 80), especially when ventricular repolarization and auricular depolarization takes place almost simultaneously.

3. *Lengthening of the P–R interval,* as seen in partial AV block, causes the P wave to become superimposed on the preceding T wave, as in figure 81.

4. In *auricular fibrillation,* depolarization of the auricle is greatly altered, and no definite P waves can be seen (Fig. 82).

5. In *auricular premature contractions* originating from a site in the auricles near the atrioventricular valves, or in retrograde conduction from the AV node, the P wave is inverted in leads II and III (Fig. 83). Consult the chapter on Disturbances in Cardiac Mechanism for further details concerning changes in the P wave due to disturbance in cardiac mechanism.

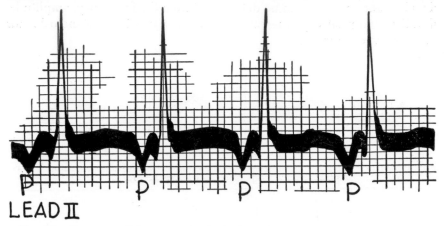

LEAD II

FIG. 83.—Inversion of the P wave in lead II in AV nodal rhythm with retrograde conduction.

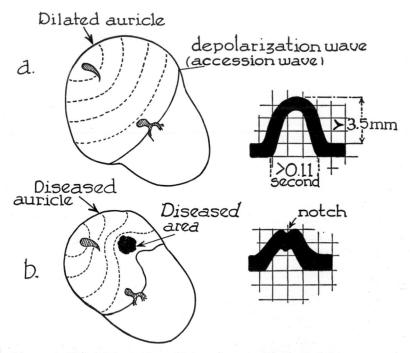

FIG. 84.—*a*, A dilated left auricle produces a P wave of increased duration. *b*, Local variations in disease produce deformity of the P wave.

6. *Sinus tachycardia*, regardless of its cause (exercise, emotion, thyrotoxicosis) tends to produce high peaked P waves (Fig. 79).

In *patients with mitral stenosis* the left auricle is often enlarged and diseased. If the auricle is hypertrophied and *dilated*, the duration of the depolarization process will be increased, and the P wave will be wide. If the auricles are *diseased* as well, the migration of the depolarization process may be retarded and further widening of the P wave will ensue. If there are *localized areas of disease*, the depolarization process will take place in an irregular manner and the P wave will be notched, slurred or deformed in some way. If an auricle is *hypertrophied*, the amplitude of the wave will be increased, as the amplitude tends to vary directly with the mass of the muscle depolarized (Fig. 84).

THE P–R (P–Q) INTERVAL

The P–R interval extends from the beginning of the P wave to the beginning of the Q or R wave of the QRS complex. Some cardiologists speak of the P–Q interval (see next paragraph) when the first wave of the QRS complex is a Q wave instead of an R wave. It is customary, however, to use the term P–R interval regardless of the initial wave of the QRS complex. The upper limit of normal for cardiac rates above 70 beats per minute is *0.20 second* (see Appendix, Table 3, for details). A P–R interval greater than 0.20 second for cardiac rates greater than 70 beats per minute is evidence of partial atrioventricular block, a definite sign of cardiac disease. The P–R interval is a measure of the time required to depolarize the auricular musculature plus the delay in the AV node plus the time required to depolarize enough ventricular muscle to produce sufficient current to begin the QRS complex. The P–R interval varies with body size and cardiac rate. Thus, if a patient has a cardiac rate of 100 beats per minute and a P–R interval of 0.20 second, he has evidence of partial AV block or cardiac disease, since the upper limit of normal for a cardiac rate of 100 is *0.18 second* (see Appendix, Table 3).

The P–R interval may, in rare instances, exceed the upper limit of normal in individuals with no apparent disease. Diphtheria, acute rheumatic fever, congenital anomalies of the junctional tissue, arteriosclerosis, syphilitic heart disease, and coronary occlusion, particularly of the right coronary artery, frequently prolong the P–R interval. In fact, any disease which produces changes in the AV node or bundle of His may produce a prolonged P–R interval. Digitalis may also lengthen the interval.

It is well to remember that the width of the P wave influences the duration of the P–R interval. Therefore, disease of the auricular musculature likewise will cause prolongation of the P–R interval. The relative contributions made by impairment of conduction of the impulse in the auricle or junctional tissues may be estimated by the relative prolongations of the P wave and P–R segment (see next paragraph).

THE P–R (P–Q) SEGMENT

The P–R segment is measured from the end of the P wave to the beginning of the QRS complex. Since the depolarization process of the auricles reaches the AV node a moment after the peak of the P wave is inscribed, the segment plus the latter portion of the P wave represents the length of time required for migration of the impulse through the junc-

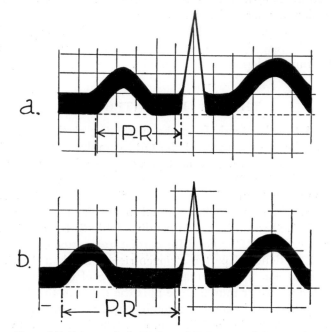

Fig. 85.—*a*, Normal P–R interval. *b*, Prolonged P–R interval (incomplete AV block).

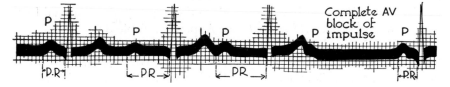

Fig. 86.—Partial AV block of the Wenckebach type, illustrating the successive lengthening of the P–R interval and the "dropped" QRS complex.

tional tissues to the ventricular muscle. The normal range for the segment length is from *0.02 to 0.12 second*. Lengthening of this segment is indicative of disease of the AV node or bundle of His.

A diagnosis of *incomplete AV block* is made when the P–R interval exceeds the upper limit of normal (Fig. 85). There are unlimited degrees of partial AV block. In rare instances the P–R interval may measure as much as 1.0 second. Slight prolongation of the P–R interval represents a slight degree of AV block.

A special type of partial AV block, sometimes referred to as the *Wenckebach periods or phenomena*, occurs when the P–R interval increases in length with each successive cardiac cycle until the impulse, originating in the SA node, is completely blocked at the AV node and fails to initiate a QRS complex. When the impulse fails to pass through the AV node, a QRS complex does not follow the P wave. Because of this extra period of rest and because the AV node is nonrefractory, the next P–R

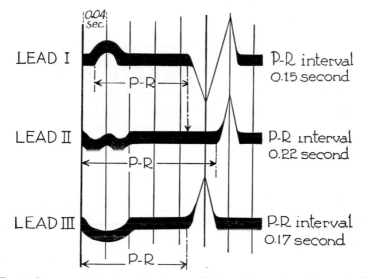

FIG. 87.—A diagram of the three leads recorded simultaneously. The vertical arrow indicates the beginning of Q_2. (See text for explanations.)

interval again appears short, and the successive P–R intervals lengthen as the AV node becomes more refractory until finally another QRS complex fails to follow the P wave. This cycle of events is continuously repeated (Fig. 86).

It is usually stated that the P–R interval should be measured in lead II. That such a rule may result in errors in measurement is demonstrated by figure 87. For example, in lead II (Fig. 87) the P–R interval measures 0.22 second and is therefore abnormally long and indicative of AV block and cardiac disease. However, close examination reveals that an isoelectric Q wave in lead II was included with the P–R interval, which, of course, is erroneous. That an isoelectric Q_2 is present is evidenced by the fact that according to Einthoven's law $Q_1 + Q_3 = Q_2$, and since Q_1 is negative, Q_3 must be positive and Q_2 zero or isoelectric.

It can also be seen in figure 87 that the first part of P_1 is isoelectric; therefore the P–R interval in lead I is too short and does not represent the true measurement. The P–R interval in lead III in the electrocardiogram shown in figure 87 is the correct one to measure; this is seen to be 0.17 second and is therefore within normal limits.

It is very simple to make such measurements when the leads are recorded simultaneously. Under ordinary clinical circumstances, when each lead is recorded successively, it is necessary to use judgment to avoid errors in measurements. *The best rule to follow is to choose a lead for analysis in which there is a well formed, wide P wave and a prominent Q wave, or if there is no Q wave in the lead, the measurement should be made in the lead with the widest QRS complex.*

THE AURICULAR T WAVE

Just as the depolarization wave of the ventricle is followed by a repolarization wave, the T wave, so is the auricular depolarization wave followed by a wave of auricular repolarization which is called the *auricular T wave*. Clinically, the auricular T wave is not of great significance today. However, its recognition is important in certain isolated instances:

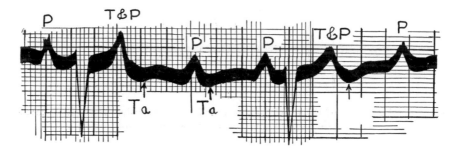

Fɪɢ. 88.—Complete heart block showing the auricular T wave. Ta = auricular T wave.

1. Its presence helps in identifying P waves in certain types of disturbances in cardiac mechanism (Fig. 88), and

2. It occasionally produces depression of a portion of the S–T segment, which should not be considered abnormal (Fig. 89).

Generally, the auricular T wave is not seen, as it is either small or falls completely within the QRS complex. The shift of the S–T or P–R interval produced by the auricular T wave is rarely more than a fraction of a millimeter. It is to be noted that the normal auricular T wave is opposite in direction to the P wave, whereas the normal ventricular T wave is usually deflected in the same direction as the major deflection of the QRS complex.

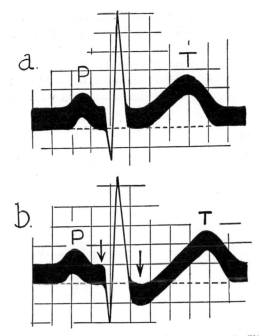

FIG. 89.—*a*, Tracing showing no visible auricular T wave. *b*, Slight depression of the S–T segment caused by ventricular depolarization occurring simultaneously with auricular repolarization.

THE QRS COMPLEX

The QRS complex is measured from the beginning of the Q or R wave to the end of the R or S wave. The duration of the complex should be measured in the *limb lead* in which it is greatest, in order to avoid any errors due to isoelectric portions of the QRS complex at its beginning or termination. The beginning of the complex represents the beginning of ventricular depolarization and the end of the complex indicates the completion of ventricular depolarization. Two factors which increase the duration of the QRS complex are: (1) decrease in the rate of depolarization, such as is encountered in disease of the myocardium; and (2) increase in the distance traveled by the depolarization wave, as in ventricular hypertrophy.

The QRS complex may assume many shapes, some of which are illustrated in figure 90.

The *normal range* for the QRS interval for adults is from *0.06 to 0.10 second*. In the younger age groups it ranges from 0.045 in infants to 0.09 in older children. It is rare for the QRS complex to be less than 0.06 second in the adult. A duration greater than 0.10 second is *usually evidence of cardiac disease* and indicates depression of the rate of ventricular depolarization. The duration of the complex varies with the cardiac rate

6

and with the height of the patient. The more rapid the rate and the shorter the patient, as in children, the shorter the duration of the QRS complex. Thus, with rapid rates, such as are seen in patients with auricular tachycardia, a duration of 0.09 second or even less may be abnormal. *Quinidine* increases the duration somewhat, but digitalis has essentially no effect on its duration other than that associated with changes in cardiac rate.

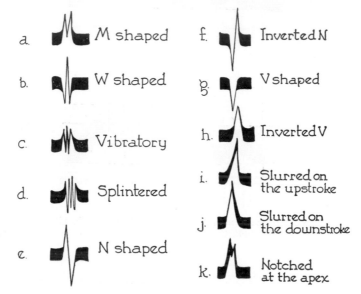

a. M shaped
b. W shaped
c. Vibratory
d. Splintered
e. N shaped
f. Inverted N
g. V shaped
h. Inverted V
i. Slurred on the upstroke
j. Slurred on the downstroke
k. Notched at the apex

FIG. 90.—Various normal configurations of the QRS complex. The first four forms occur frequently in lead III.

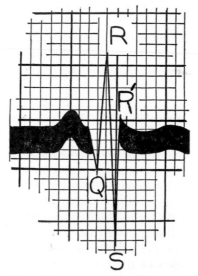

FIG. 91.—The waves of the QRS complex.

The various waves which constitute the QRS complex are the Q, R, S and R prime (R′) waves.

1. The *Q wave* may be defined as the downward deflection which initiates the QRS complex.

2. The *R wave* is defined as the initial upward deflection.

3. The *S wave* is defined as the initial downward deflection following the R wave.

4. The R′ (R prime) wave, which follows the S wave (Fig. 91), is described as the second positive deflection. A negative wave occurring im-

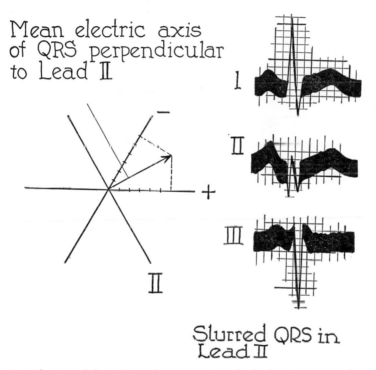

Mean electric axis
of QRS perpendicular
to Lead II

Slurred QRS in
Lead II

Fig. 92.—Slurring of the QRS tends to occur in a lead when the mean electric axis of the QRS complex is perpendicular to the respective lead line. This is shown in lead II.

mediately after the R′ wave is the S′ wave, the successive positive and negative deflections being labeled R″, S″, R‴, S‴, etc. As a general rule, the deflections are not labeled beyond the R′ wave.

The above definitions are empiric and with experience will be found to be inadequate.

Slurring occurs normally to some extent at the beginning of the upstroke and at the apex of the waves as the string is moving relatively slowly or is changing its direction of movement at these moments. Slurring also tends to take place normally in a lead whenever the mean electric axis of the QRS complex tends to be perpendicular to the respective lead line of the triaxial reference system (Fig. 92).

In *disease of the muscle of the ventricles,* slurring, notching, and abnormal configurations of the QRS complex occur because the depolarization process takes place in an irregular or abnormal manner. These abnormal configurations of the QRS complex are *not specific for any disease entity* but may be produced by any disease which disturbs the ventricular musculature or Purkinje system morphologically or functionally in such a way as to interfere with the order of depolarization.

The amplitude of the QRS complex in at least one of the three standard leads should normally measure more than 5 millimeters (0.5 millivolts). Amplitudes of 5 millimeters or less suggest the presence of cardiac disease (Fig. 93).

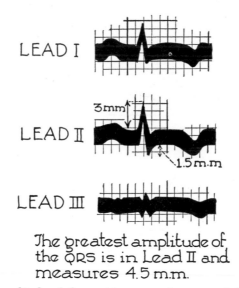

LEAD I

LEAD II

3mm

1.5 m.m

LEAD III

The greatest amplitude of the QRS is in Lead II and measures 4.5 m.m.

Fig. 93.—The amplitude of the positive waves is measured from the top of the isoelectric line to the top of the highest upward deflection. This is added, without regard to sign, to a measurement of the deepest downward deflection, which is measured from the bottom of the isoelectric line to the apex of the deepest deflection. The sum of these two represents the amplitude of the QRS complex. Corrections for the width of the string are made when measurements are obtained in this manner.

THE Q WAVE

The Q wave is usually not greater than 3 millimeters in depth in leads I and II and, as a rule, varies between 0 and 1 millimeter. This Q wave is due to depolarization of the septum. A larger Q wave may be found in lead III or in other leads, but these large Q waves are not septal in origin. The Q wave may be found normally in any lead. The duration of the Q wave usually does not exceed 0.03 second. When a Q wave is present in lead I, it is also present in the precordial leads recorded from the left of the septum (*vide infra*). This rule aids in detecting technical errors in making recordings.

THE R WAVE

The highest R wave in any of the three standard leads normally varies between 4 and 22 *millimeters* or 0.4 and 2.2 millivolts. The duration is seldom greater than *0.07 second*. The upper limits may be exceeded in patients with cardiac hypertrophy or dilatation or with cardiac disease of many sorts.

THE S WAVE

The upper limit of normal for the amplitude of the S wave for any lead in adults is 6 *millimeters*. S waves may be found in all three leads normally, or they may be absent from any or all of the standard leads.

BUNDLE BRANCH BLOCK

In the foregoing discussion it was pointed out that disease of the auricular muscle often produces abnormally shaped P waves, with widening of the wave, and that disease of the AV node or bundle of His may be responsible for a type of block which manifests itself as a prolongation of the P–R segment. When disease occurs in the branches of the bundle of

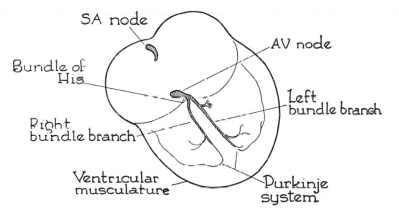

Fig. 94.—Diagram of the conduction system of the heart.

His and delays conduction, the condition is spoken of as bundle branch block and it manifests itself as a prolongation of the QRS interval. It is obvious at a glance that disease may involve either the right or left bundle branch and that there may be either complete or incomplete inhibition of the transmission of the impulse. The block may occur in the *bundles themselves* or in the *Purkinje network* (arborization block). Inhibition of depolarization of the *ventricular muscle* as the process passes from the Purkinje system to the epicardium is often called *defective intra-ventricular conduction* (Fig. 94).

Classification of Bundle Branch Block

Bundle branch block (BBB) has been classified variously. For the sake of simplicity and until there is sufficient clinical evidence accumulated to warrant a more detailed classification, the following one is suggested:

I. Complete Bundle Branch Block
  A. Left
    1. Typical
    2. Atypical
  B. Right
    1. Typical
    2. Atypical
II. Incomplete Bundle Branch Block (arborization block and defective intraventricular conduction)
  A. Left
  B. Right
III. Paroxysmal (Transitory) Bundle Branch Block
    This may include a paroxysm of variable length of any of the above types.
IV. Partial Bundle Branch Block
    This includes a block of any of the above types alternating in a 2:1, 3:1, 3:2, etc., ratio with normal conductions.
V. False Bundle Branch Block (Bundle of Kent syndrome, Wolff-Parkinson-White syndrome or pre-excitation syndrome).

I. Complete Bundle Branch Block.—This is present whenever the impulse migrating down from the AV node through the bundle of His is completely obstructed by a lesion in the left or right bundle, so that its passage directly to the Purkinje system is prevented.

Diagnostic Criteria.—Two criteria are necessary to make the diagnosis electrocardiographically: (1) The QRS complexes must be greater than 0.12 second in duration in any or all standard leads for a normal resting cardiac rate. Necessary allowance must be made for more rapid cardiac rates. (2) It is necessary to make sure that the impulse traveled along the usual path in reaching the bundles in order to avoid errors which might occur because of ventricular premature beats. The P waves and the P–R intervals preceding the QRS complexes assure the usual order of migration of the impulse to the bundles.

A. Complete Left Bundle Branch Block.—Obviously, once a diagnosis of BBB (the abbreviation which will be used henceforth for bundle branch block) has been established, it is advisable to determine whether passage of impulses through the left or right bundle has been obstructed. In order to determine the bundle involved, it is necessary that the block must have been present when lead I was recorded or during the recording of the precordial leads. (The rôle of the precordial leads will be discussed in Chapter 3.) It is *not possible* to localize the bundle involved from lead II or lead III.

Diagnostic Criterion.—When the main deflection of the QRS complex is up, or positive, in lead I, left complete BBB is present. By *main* deflection is meant that of greatest *duration* and not necessarily of greatest amplitude. This deflection usually is much deformed by slurring and notching (Fig. 95).

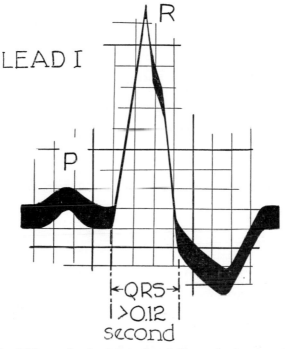

Fig. 95.—The QRS complex is greater than 0.12 sec. in duration and the impulse traveled to the bundles by the normal path, as shown by the P wave and P–R segment, thus indicating *complete BBB*. The main deflection of the QRS complex in lead I is up, or positive; therefore, it is *left complete BBB*.

Mechanisms.—It can be seen from figure 96 why the *main deflection, i.e.,* the one of greatest duration, is *up, or positive, in lead I* and is usually deformed. The impulse coming down through the AV node and bundle of His enters the right and left bundle branches. Because of the lesion in the left bundle branch, the impulse cannot pass through. It does pass through the right branch and is rapidly distributed by the Purkinje system to the subendocardial layer of the right ventricular muscle. The depolarization process rapidly depolarizes the right ventricular muscle (arrows *a* and *b*, Fig. 96). Because of the anterior position of the right ventricle and the concomitant depolarization of the septum neutralizing the force of depolarization of the free wall of the right ventricle, the resultant depolarization process produces little electric effect upon the *RA* and *LA* electrodes in lead I. The depolarization process then reaches the left ventricle through the septum (dotted arrow *c*, Fig. 96) and the subendocardial surfaces and the Purkinje system. The impulse is then rapidly distributed by the Purkinje fibers on the left, distal to the lesion in the left bundle, to the subendocardial layer of muscle of the left ventricle. The depolarization process then migrates outward to the epicardium of the left ventricle (arrow *d*, Fig. 96). The forces represented by arrows *c* and

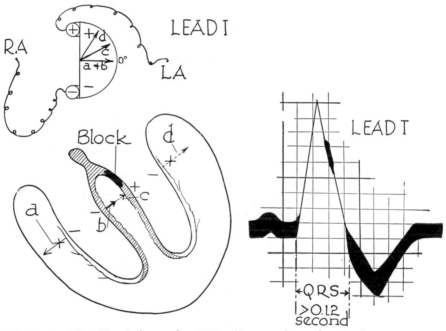

Fig. 96.—Left complete BBB. (See text for explanation.)

d are unbalanced and produce an upward deflection in lead I. Thus, it can be seen that the abnormal roundabout course of the depolarization process is slow (requiring about 0.04 sec. to traverse the septum alone) and mainly from right to left, producing a field of relative negativity for the *RA* electrode and relative positivity for the *LA* electrode. This, as previously stated in Chapter 1, causes a wide upright or positive deflection in lead I. The abnormal course is responsible for the *slurring and notching* or *abnormal* configuration of the upright or *positive* deflection.

1. *Typical Complete Left BBB.—Diagnostic Criteria.—*If the criteria for *complete left BBB* are present (see immediately preceding) and if (1) the main (greatest duration) deflection of the QRS is up in lead I and down in lead III, and (2) the T waves in leads I and III are opposite

in direction to the main deflections of the QRS, then the left complete BBB is *typical*. Any variations from these criteria indicate *atypical left complete BBB* (Fig. 97).

The classification of complete BBB into *typical* and *atypical* is purely empiric, the significance of which is unknown. Differences are most likely attributable to variations in the order of the repolarization process, although disturbances in the order of depolarization or in cardiac position may also contribute.

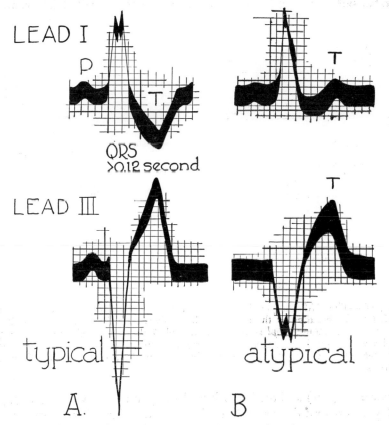

Fɪɢ. 97.—Typical and atypical left complete bundle branch block. The block is atypical in B because T_1 is not opposite to the main deflections of QRS_1.

B. **Complete Right Bundle Branch Block.**—*Diagnostic Criterion.*— When the main deflection (the one of greatest duration) of the QRS complex is down in lead I, *right complete BBB* is present. Of course, as for left complete BBB, it is necessary to make certain that the criterion for complete BBB is present and that the impulse has reached the bundle branches by means of the usual path. The main deflection in right complete BBB is usually greatly deformed (Fig. 98).

Mechanisms.—It can be seen from figure 99 why the main deflection of the QRS is *down* in lead I in right complete BBB and why it is usually deformed. The impulse traveling down through the AV node and the bundle of His enters the right and left bundle branches. Because of the lesion in the right branch, the impulse is completely blocked and therefore is unable to pass through that bundle. It continues through the left bundle branch, however, and is rapidly distributed to the subendocardial layer of muscle in the left ventricle. There the depolarization process migrates out to the epicardial surface of the thick-walled left ventricle

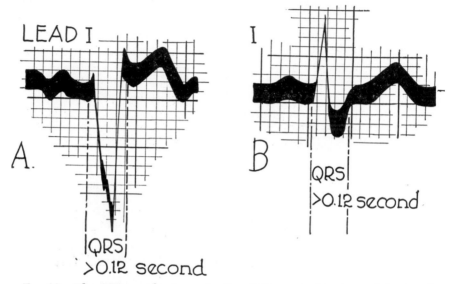

Fɪɢ. 98.—The QRS complex is greater than 0.12 sec. in duration and the impulse traveled to the bundles by the normal path, as shown by the P wave and P–R segment, thus indicating *complete BBB.* In A and B the main deflection of the QRS complex is down in lead I; therefore it is *right complete BBB.* Note in B the downward deflection is of *greatest duration* but the upright deflection is of greatest amplitude.

(arrow *a*, Fig. 99) and the left half of the septum (arrow *b*, Fig. 99), producing an upward deflection in lead I. The depolarization process in the septum (arrow *c*, Fig. 99) continues through until it reaches the right Purkinje system. The impulse is then rapidly distributed by the Purkinje fibers throughout the subendocardial layer of muscle of the right ventricle. The depolarization process continues out to the epicardial surface of the right ventricular musculature (arrow *d*, Fig. 99). It can be seen, therefore, that the latter part of the depolarization of the ventricular musculature is from left to right and slow and abnormal in its course. This results in a *prolonged deformed downward* deflection. The deflection is down in lead I because the *LA* electrode is in a field of relative negativity most of the time, whereas the *RA* electrode is in a field of relative positivity during the slow latter part of the depolarization of the muscle of the right ventricle.

In right BBB, because of the large mass of muscle in the free wall of the left ventricle and because of the relative position of this ventricle, the early phase of depolarization results in the overneutralization of the early depolarization process in the septum moving from left to right ventricle. This produces a normal-appearing upward deflection in lead I. This early depolarization process in the left ventricle and left half of the septum is soon completed, leaving the depolarization process moving from left to right through the septum and leaving the free wall of the right ventricle unbalanced, and thus making the left arm electrode relatively negative and the right arm electrode relatively positive. A wide slurred downward deflection of the terminal portion of the QRS complex in lead I results.

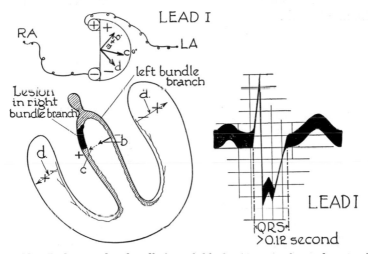

FIG. 99.—Right complete bundle branch block. (See text for explanation.)

1. *Typical Right Complete BBB.—Diagnostic Criteria.*—If the criteria for complete right BBB are present (see immediately preceding) and if (1) the main deflection of the QRS complex (one of greatest duration) is down in lead I and up in lead III, and (2) the T waves are opposite in direction to the main deflections of the QRS in these leads, the right complete BBB is *typical.* Any variations from these criteria indicate *atypical* right complete BBB (Fig. 100).

II. **Incomplete Bundle Branch Block.**—As stated previously, the *normal* QRS complex does not exceed 0.10 second and in *complete* BBB the QRS complex is greater than 0.12 second at the normal resting cardiac rate. QRS intervals greater than 0.10 second but not exceeding 0.12 second may be produced by *incomplete BBB.* If there is a normal electric axis of the QRS and the QRS interval is greater than 0.10 but not greater than 0.12 second, then the tracing is interpreted as indicating *defective* *intraventricular conduction, i.e.,* probably disturbances in conduction in the ventricular musculature. There is usually some slurring and notching of the QRS complexes. If the tracing resembles right or left complete BBB but the QRS complex is not over 0.12 second in width, a diagnosis of *incomplete right or left bundle branch block* is made, *i.e.,* disturbances in conduction but not complete blocking of impulses in the main bundle branches. When the QRS complexes tend to be low in amplitude, the term *arborization block* is used, suggesting defective conduction in the smaller branches of the Purkinje system. It is well to note that the syndrome "arborization block" is arbitrary and therefore subject to controversy. Consult figure 101 for illustrations.

Hypertrophy of the crista supraventricularis produces relatively wide, slurred S waves in leads I, V_5 and V_6 (see Chapter 3). These prominent S waves are often mistaken to reflect delayed conduction through the right bundle branch.

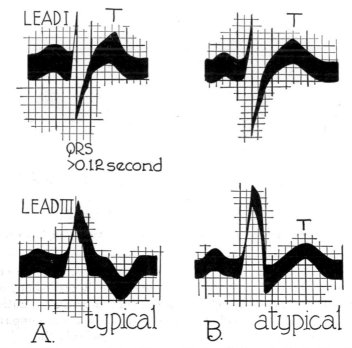

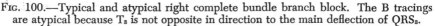

Fig. 100.—Typical and atypical right complete bundle branch block. The B tracings are atypical because T_3 is not opposite in direction to the main deflection of QRS_3.

The QRS interval may reach 0.12 second when there is severe hypertrophy of the ventricular wall. This prolongation of the QRS complex is due to the greater distance over which the depolarization process must travel in order to traverse the thickened wall of the ventricle completely. Under such circumstances the QRS complex has a normal configuration, since the order of the process of depolarization is essentially normal and the intrinsic deflection is delayed (see Chapter 3).

III. Paroxysmal Bundle Branch Block.—When the block occurs in successive showers or paroxysms, which last from periods of a few beats to hours or longer, alternating with periods of normal conduction, the picture is referred to as *paroxysmal or transitory BBB* (Fig. 102).

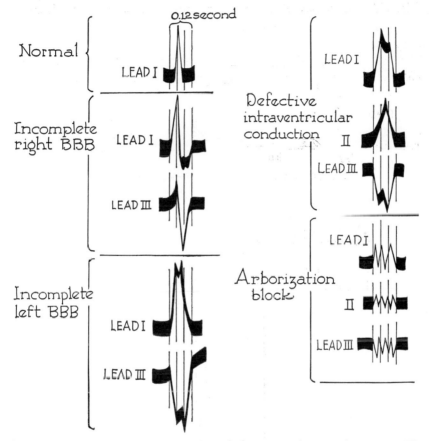

FIG. 101.—Diagrammatic representation of the types of *incomplete BBB*. The duration of the QRS complexes in all the above illustrations is *greater than* 0.10 second but *not greater than* 0.12 second.

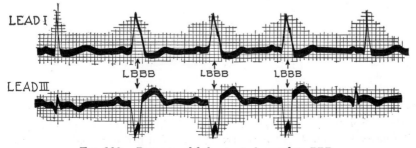

FIG. 102.—Paroxysmal left atypical complete BBB.

IV. Partial Bundle Branch Block.—Partial bundle branch block is an uncommon type of BBB. If there is one normal QRS complex alternating with one block complex, the block is designated as 2:1 partial BBB. If there is one normal QRS complex with two block complexes, the block is designated as 3:1 block. A 3:2 or 4:3 block, and so forth, may occur (Fig. 103). One may distinguish ventricular premature beats from BBB

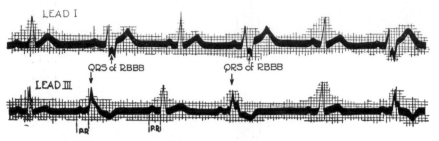

Fig. 103.—A 2:1 partial right typical complete BBB.

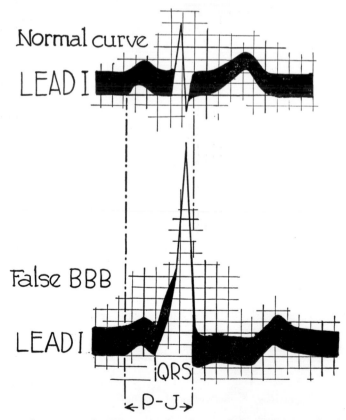

Fig. 104.—False BBB. The P–R interval is short and the QRS interval is long. The P–J interval is normal. There is slurring of the first part of the QRS complex.
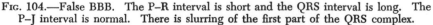

(see Chapter 4) by observing the absence of a P wave or shortening of the P–R interval in the latter case.

Obviously, the complexes of any of the types of block previously dis-cussed under *complete BBB* or *incomplete BBB* may alternate with the normal complex. The term applied to the block is determined by the type of block indicated by the abnormal complex.

Clinical Significance of Bundle Branch Block.—The four groups of BBB described may be produced by any type of cardiac disease which is asso-ciated with a lesion of the bundle branches or their subdivisions. For

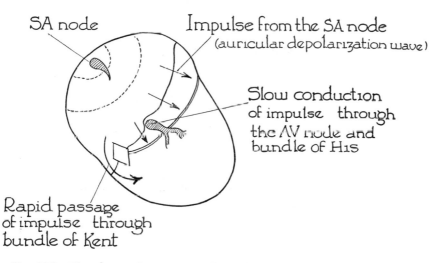

FIG. 105.—The abnormal connection of muscle between the auricle and ventricle (bundle of Kent) with the early transmission of the impulse through the bundle of Kent.

example, a rheumatic nodule (Aschoff body), a gumma, infarct, or neo-plastic lesion of the right or left bundle branch will produce right or left BBB respectively. The tendency is for clinical states which are respon-sible for left ventricular hypertrophy and disease to produce *left BBB* and for those which cause right ventricular hypertrophy and disease to pro-duce *right BBB*. Posterior infarcts are more apt to produce BBB, since the two bundles usually receive their blood supply from branches of the pos-terior or right coronary artery. Any of the four types of BBB indicate *definite* evidence of cardiac disease, *regardless* of the other clinical cardiac findings. Remember, however, that the mere finding of a BBB does not mean impending death, for many patients live a long time with it. In gen-eral, the prognosis is worse in left BBB than in right BBB. Never include a statement of prognosis in the routine interpretaion of electrocardiogram.

V. False Bundle Branch Block (Bundle of Kent Syndrome).—False bundle branch block is usually referred to as the *Wolff-Parkinson-White syndrome*, the *bundle of Kent syndrome*, or *pre-excitation syndrome*. It is important to distinguish the four types of bundle branch block discussed above from false bundle branch block, as the former four indicate

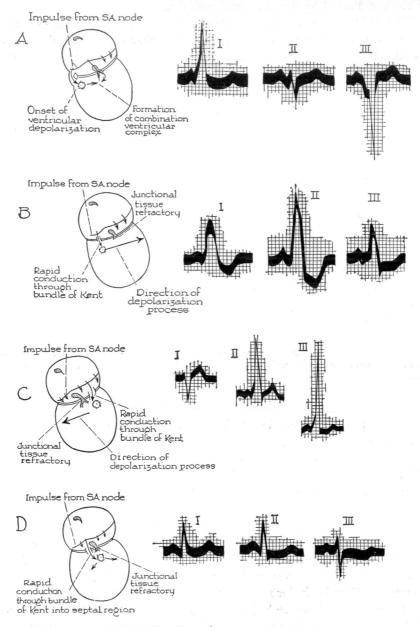

FIG. 106.—Legend on opposite page.

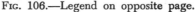

the presence of cardiac disease whereas the latter is *said to be* functional and is not ordinarily indicative of organic cardiac disease. The syndrome, however, may result in death.

Diagnostic Criteria.—A diagnosis of false BBB is made when the following findings are present: (1) The P–R interval is short (it is usually less than 0.11 second), and (2) the QRS complex is wide (it is usually 0.11 to 0.14 second). Usually, the P–R interval decreases by the amount the QRS complex lengthens, so the P–J interval remains normal.

The upstroke of the R wave in lead I is usually slurred and the S wave in lead III (if the QRS in this lead is mainly an S wave) is sometimes wide (Fig. 104), *i.e.*, the first part of the QRS complex is slurred and notched, whereas the latter part is usually normal in appearance. The reasons for this finding and the other diagnostic criteria may be explained by figure 105.

This syndrome is most commonly seen in young subjects who have frequent attacks of supraventricular tachycardia. The wide complexes sometimes disappear after exercise or the use of atropine.

FIG. 106.—Variations in the QRS configuration in Wolff-Parkinson-White syndrome. Since the aberrant bundle of conduction tissue delivers an impulse early to the ventricular musculature, a process of depolarization is initiated at the terminus of the bundle. This process of depolarization tends to influence the configuration of the electrocardiogram in a manner similar to that in which an excitation wave of depolarization process of a ventricular premature contraction influences the electrocardiographic pattern (Chapter 4). The order of this depolarization from the aberrant bundle and its time relationship with the process initiated by an impulse delivered to the ventricle by way of the Purkinje system are the important factors which determine the QRS configuration. Combination ventricular depolarization complexes usually result. For example:

A. A process of depolarization is initiated in the right ventricle by an aberrant bundle terminating there. Because of its direction and order of migration, a positive and usually slurred deflection is inscribed early in lead I. The remainder of the QRS complex is normal, because the ventricular depolarization is completed by the impulse entering through the normal pathways. A combination of these two processes of depolarization results in a combination QRS complex.

B. The process of depolarization initiated at the terminus of the aberrant bundle was responsible for the entire depolarization of the ventricular musculature. The impulse approaching from the auricles through the normal pathways was not able to enter the ventricles, since they were made refractory by the impulse originating through the aberrant bundle. Because of the direction of spread, the QRS complexes in the standard leads resemble those of multiple right ventricular premature contractions or complete left bundle branch block.

C. The depolarization process initiated at the terminus of the aberrant bundle in the left ventricle migrates from left to right. If the impulse, approaching through the normal pathways, did not enter the ventricle, this would produce QRS configurations in the standard leads similar to those of multiple left ventricular premature contractions or complete right bundle branch block.

D. The depolarization process is initiated by an impulse delivered by way of an aberrant bundle into the septum or in or near the bundle of His. The P–R interval is short, and the QRS complex is only slightly, if at all, prolonged and is deformed relatively little, since the order of depolarization is not particularly abnormal. Such a situation is difficult to identify unless the impulse enters by way of the normal pathways from time to time.

7

It is thought that the short P–R interval can be explained by an abnormal muscular communication, the bundle of Kent, or band of conduction tissue between an auricle and a ventricle. The impulses from the SA node travel more rapidly through the bundle of Kent than through the AV node and bundle of His. The widening of the QRS complex and the slurring of the R wave are explained by the depolarization process entering the ventricle early and without any delay through the abnormal connection between the auricle and ventricle (Fig. 105), which makes the P–R interval short. Since the course of the impulse is abnormal and early during depolarization of the ventricle, the early part of the QRS complex is slurred or notched. Also, since the depolarization process continues over a longer period of time than normally, the QRS complex is exceptionally wide. After the depolarization process of the ventricle, initiated by the impulse entering through the bundle of Kent, is partially under way, the impulse that was previously delayed at the AV node now enters the ventricle by the normal path, and the depolarization of the ventricles is finally completed in normal fashion.

This concept of "pre-excitation" of the ventricles by means of a bundle of Kent can also be explained in the following manner. It is possible that if a highly sensitive area existed in the ventricular musculature, contraction of the atria could tug sufficiently on the ventricles and initiate an impulse (a late premature or ectopic beat) that would start a wave of polarization in the ventricle before the impulse traveling through the normal conducting pathways had time to enter the ventricles to complete depolarization.

It is obvious, however, that although the description outlined of the electrocardiographic configuration for the Wolff-Parkinson-White syndrome is of the type most frequently encountered, variations in the configuration do occur. A detailed discussion of these variations will not be attempted here, but it is not difficult to predict or identify them. One has merely to realize that the QRS complex in the Wolff-Parkinson-White syndrome is the result of a process of ventricular depolarization initiated at an ectopic focus, for example, at the terminus of the aberrant conduction tissue, with or without the algebraic addition of the electric forces of another process of ventricular depolarization initiated from an impulse delivered through the normal pathways (junctional tissues). The process of depolarization originating through the aberrant pathway would tend to produce a configuration of the QRS complex similar to that observed in a premature beat originating at the same site in the ventricle (Chapter 4). Thus, there may be combination of ventricular complexes (Chapter 4) to which the depolarization processes from the normal and aberrant pathways contribute to a variable degree. Occasionally, the former does not contribute at all, as in the case when the depolarization process originating from the aberrant tissue produces complete refraction of the ventricular muscle when the normal impulse is about to enter the ventricles. Figure 106 illustrates several variations in the configurations.

It is well to note that if there are several aberrant bundles of tissue which bring about electric connections between the atria and ventricles, an equal number of depolarization processes may cause electric forces which combine algebraically to produce a QRS complex.

The bundle of Kent is said to predispose to attacks of paroxysmal tachycardia by facilitating retrograde conduction into the auricle with the initiation of circus movements or an abnormal mechanism, such as supraventricular tachycardia.

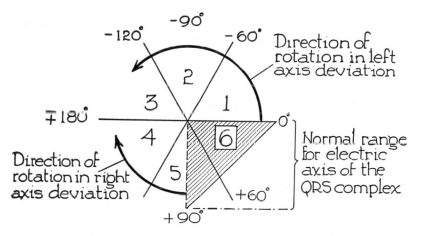

FIG. 107.—The triaxial reference system showing the sextants and the range of the normal axis of the QRS complex as well as the direction of rotation in left or right axis deviation.

THE MEAN ELECTRIC AXIS OF THE DEPOLARIZATION PROCESS OF THE VENTRICLES

The method for determining the direction of the mean electric axis of the QRS complex—the depolarization wave of the ventricles—from the electrocardiogram by means of the triaxial reference system has been presented (Chapter 1). The direction of the mean electric axis of the depolarization process is expressed as a deviation of the axis in degrees (minus or plus, that is, counterclockwise or clockwise deviation, respectively), from the three o'clock axis (lead I line) of the triaxial reference system. It may also be expressed as falling into any one of the six sextants of the triaxial reference system (Figs. 107 and 285). There are *three types of axis deviations* for the QRS complex: (1) *normal axis deviation* is present when the electric axis is between 0 and +90 degrees; (2) *right axis deviation* is present when the electric axis is to the right, or more positive than +90 degrees, and (3) *left axis deviation* is present when the axis is to the left, or more negative than 0 degree (Fig. 107).

The Normal Mean Electric Axis of the QRS Complex

The direction of the mean normal electric axis varies considerably with the age of the subject. In the *infant* under six months of age, the axis is greatly to the right (+130 degrees). *Between the ages of one and five years* the axis moves to the left, the average for these ages inclusive being

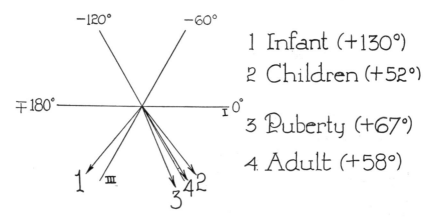

1 Infant (+130°)

2 Children (+52°)

3 Puberty (+67°)

4 Adult (+58°)

Fig. 108.—Changes in direction of the mean electric axis of the QRS complex with age in normal human subjects.

about +52 degrees. The axis then returns to the right at *puberty,* the average axis being about +67 degrees. It again returns to the left in the *adult,* averaging about +58 degrees (Fig. 108). These changes in position are due mainly to the changing position of the heart in the thorax, except in the case of the infant.

Right Axis Deviation

Right axis deviation is characterized by an S_1 that is of greater amplitude than R_1 and by an R_3 that is higher than R_1 or R_2 (Fig. 109).

Right axis deviation usually indicates *disease when the axis is more positive than +110 degrees.* A right axis deviation of *from +100 degrees to +110 degrees is strongly suggestive evidence of cardiac disease.* It is most unusual for the position of the heart in the thorax alone to produce a mean electric axis of +100 degrees or greater. Extreme right axis deviation is normal for infants up to six months of age and is attributable to fetal circulation, with the greater load on the right ventricle.

Right axis deviation may be due *normally* to: (1) a dropped heart, that is, a vertical or ptotic position of the heart in the chest, frequently seen in tall thin individuals; and (2) early infancy, as stated previously.

In *disease states* right axis deviation is due to: (1) dilatation or hypertrophy of the right ventricle, which also slightly rotates the heart clockwise on its longitudinal anatomic axis (the axis running from the center

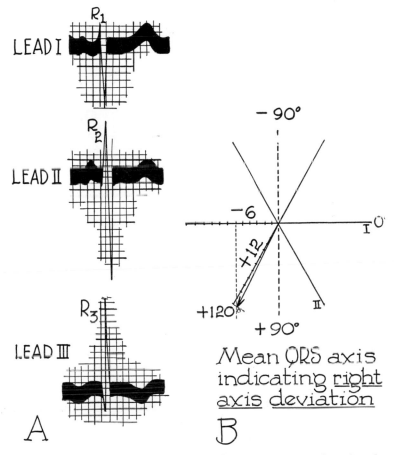

FIG. 109.—A, Right axis deviation. The avis deviation is 117° and is plotted on the triaxial reference system.

of the apex to the center of the base) as viewed from its apex, and (2), in most cases, the presence of right BBB.

Such disease states as mitral stenosis, pulmonary stenosis, pulmonary hypertension, tetralogy of Fallot, Eisenmenger syndrome, large inter-auricular septal defect and acute right ventricular failure may be associated with the electrocardiographic picture of *right axis deviation.* All factors which are responsible for strain on the right ventricle tend to bring about right axis deviation.

It is well to point out at this time that the areas under the QRS waves actually determine the mean electric axis. For practical clinical purposes, the less accurate method of employing the amplitude of the various waves of the QRS complex is used instead.

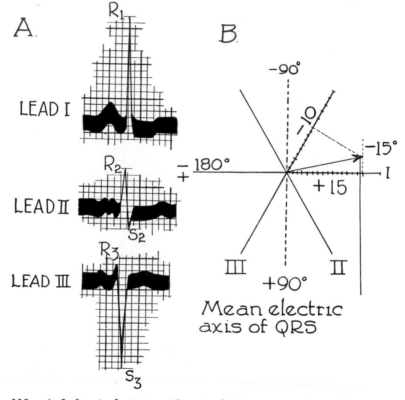

FIG. 110.—A, Left axis deviation. The axis deviation is −15° in this instance, as illustrated in the B part of the figure.

Left Axis Deviation

Left axis deviation is characterized by an S_3 that is greater in amplitude than R_3 and by an R_1 that is greater than R_2 or R_3 (Fig. 110).

In general, a left axis deviation of *from −20 to −30 degrees is strongly suggestive evidence of myocardial disease and −30 degrees or less is definite evidence of myocardial disease, with few exceptions.* To consider an electrocardiogram abnormal arbitrarily, merely upon the basis of the position of the mean electric axis of the QRS may result in error and, therefore, must be done with extreme caution, preferably after consideration of all clinical data. For example, when the apex of the normal heart is displaced posteriorly, the standard leads I, II, and III tend to have large S waves and the mean electric axis of the QRS may approach −150° in position. The QRS sÊ-loop (consult Chapter 5) is displaced backward and into the second and third sextants of the triaxial reference system in the frontal plane. Such a deviation of the electric axis is not abnormal. It is unusual for rotation of the heart to be accompanied by a mean electric axis of −20 degrees or less.

Left axis deviation is produced *normally* by a *transverse position* of the heart in the chest, as seen in hypersthenic patients, in patients with ascites, or in pregnant women.

Left axis deviation is produced by several disease states, the most important of which include:

1. *Dilatation* of the left ventricle, which rotates the heart in a counterclockwise direction about its long axis as viewed from the apex.

2. *Hypertrophy* of the left ventricle.

3. *Left bundle branch block*, complete or incomplete.

Some of the etiologic factors leading to left axis deviation are: arteriosclerotic heart disease, aortic stenosis or insufficiency, prolonged arterial hypertension, mitral insufficiency, coarctation of the aorta, acute left ventricular dilatation, prolonged arteriovenous anastomosis, anterior myocardial infarct and occasionally interventricular septal defect. All of these cause additional strain on the left ventricle. In fact, any disease state that places strain on the left ventricle will tend to produce left axis deviation.

Evaluation of Directional Deviation of the QRS Axis

It should be pointed out that although definite limits for right and left axis deviation have been set for distinguishing between the normal and abnormal heart, many factors should be considered when the direction of the electric axis of the QRS complex is evaluated. The position of the heart in the chest is of importance. Counterclockwise rotation about the long anatomic axis, as viewed from the apex, produces left axis deviation, and clockwise rotation produces right axis deviation. *Rotation of the heart about its AP axis* to the left (counterclockwise as viewed from the front), as seen in pregnant women, produces left axis deviation, and rotation to the right, as in dropped heart, produces right axis deviation. *Shifting of the mediastinum and heart* to the left tends to produce right axis deviation and a shift to the right tends to produce left axis deviation. Shifting of the mediastinum, as occurs with pneumothorax, changes the direction of the mean electric axis. This is probably effected by rotation of the heart about its axes. A heart fixed by adhesions is often not associated with a change of the electric axis of the QRS when the position of the subject is changed. In addition, the build of the patient, whether hypersthenic, hyposthenic or sthenic, the age and presence of other clinical states, such as pregnancy, are important factors to consider when the significance of apparently abnormal amounts of axis deviation is being evaluated.

Therefore, it must be remembered that, in the absence of cardiac disease, wide variations in the direction of the *mean electric axis of the QRS* may be produced by variations in position of the heart within the thorax as well as by diseases of the thorax and its contents that alter the electric conductivity of the tissues. Although the direction of the mean electric axis may be of considerable assistance in diagnosis of cardiac disease from the electrocardiogram, deviations in the axis in the absence of other electrocardiographic abnormalities must be considered cautiously.

THE MAGNITUDE OF THE MEAN ELECTRIC AXIS OF THE QRS COMPLEX

The magnitude of the mean electric axis of the QRS complex, expressed as the magnitude of a vector force, is discussed under Ventricular Gradient in Chapter 5, where QRS and gradient magnitudes are correlated.

THE JUNCTION (J)

The Junction, or J, is a site of junction between the QRS complex, usually the R or S wave, and the S–T segment or T wave (Fig. 111).

In the normal electrocardiogram J usually does not deviate from the isoelectric line by more than plus or minus 1 millimeter. This magnitude

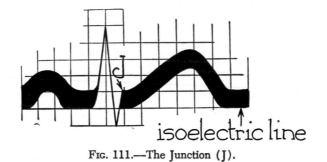

isoelectric line

Fig. 111.—The Junction (J).

of deviation is an arbitrary value. Lesser deviations may be found in patients with serious cardiac disease and greater deviations in those with normal hearts. These variations will be better appreciated after the discussions of the electrocardiographic patterns in infarction in this chapter and in Chapter 3 are consulted. When J is elevated beyond the normal limits, it is spoken of as a "high take-off" and when it is depressed, it is referred to as a "low take-off" of the S–T segment or T wave.

A high take-off may be seen in the normal heart when the repolarization process is accelerated, as in severe sinus *tachycardia* or paroxysmal supraventricular tachycardia. The junction becomes elevated because the repolarization process begins before the depolarization process has been completed (Fig. 112). This is particularly true if the terminal portion of the QRS complex is an R wave.

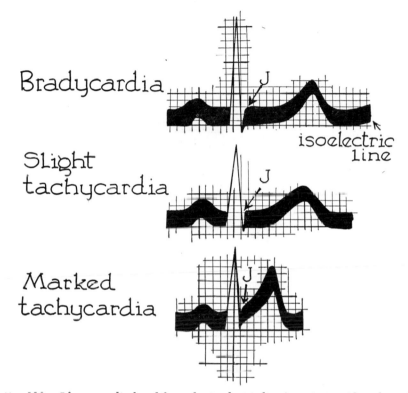

Fɪɢ. 112.—J becomes displaced from the isoelectric line in patients with tachycardia when the repolarization process (T wave) begins before the depolarization process (QRS complex) has been completed. Or stated in another way, the S–T segment shortens with an increase in cardiac rate until the segment is obliterated and the QRS complex and T wave unite directly, thus elevating J.

Electrocardiograms showing tachycardia and elevation of the junction should be retaken, if possible, after the cardiac rate is slow, to determine whether or not the shift was produced by the rapid rate or by a current of injury due to cardiac damage. This would eliminate any doubt concerning such shifts.

In the *normal heart, a low take-off* may be due to: (1) the presence of an *auricular T wave;* (2) the effect of *digitalis or related drugs;* or (3) tachycardia for reasons similar to those described above for high take-off.

When a prominent auricular T wave is present and the cardiac rate is rapid, depolarization of the ventricles often takes place simultaneously with repolarization of the auricles. When this is the case, the auricular T wave and the QRS complex are written simultaneously. As the auric-

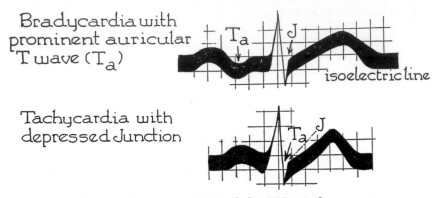

Fig. 113.—If the auricular T wave (Ta) and the QRS complex are written more or less simultaneously, as seen in patients with tachycardia, J is often depressed.

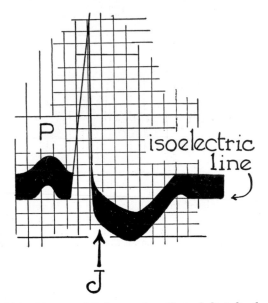

Fig. 114.—Depressed J due to the effect of digitalis therapy.

ular T wave is usually negative when the P wave is positive, a depression of the junction ensues (Fig. 113).

Following medication with digitalis and related drugs, J may be depressed along with the S–T segment in a normal heart. This is thought to be due to rapid repolarization of the ventricles (Fig. 114).

In *patients with cardiac disease,* notably those with coronary occlusion and pericarditis, the junction is abnormally displaced below or above the isoelectric line. These states will be discussed in detail below. It is well to remember that whenever the S–T segment is displaced from the iso-electric line, J is also displaced.

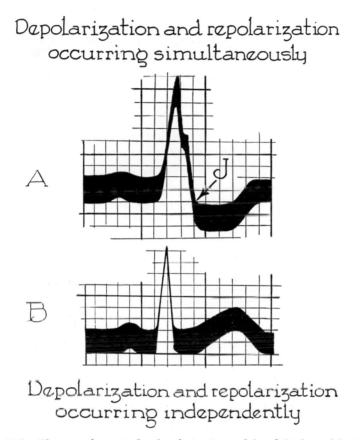

Depolarization and repolarization
occurring simultaneously

Depolarization and repolarization
occurring independently

FIG. 115.—The rate of ventricular depolarization is delayed (indicated by the wide, slurred and notched R wave in *A*) so that ventricular repolarization begins before depolarization is completed. *B* shows a QRS complex of normal width without dis-placement of J.

The disease states which produce an abnormal widening of the QRS complex may produce a displacement of J above or below the isoelectric line (Fig. 115). A delay in the rate of depolarization, so that repolariza-tion will begin before depolarization is completed, results in simultaneous depolarization and repolarization, with displacement of J. In bundle branch block or ventricular premature beats, depolarization in one ven-tricle often occurs simultaneously with repolarization in the other.

THE S–T SEGMENT

The S–T segment is measured from the end of the QRS complex to the beginning of the T wave. The duration of the segment represents, roughly, the duration of the depolarized state. The segment length varies inversely with the cardiac rate. It is longer in women than in men. The normal range for adults with a cardiac rate of 65 beats per minute measured in the lead with the shortest segment, which is usually the lead with the tallest T wave, is from 0 to 0.15 second (see Appendix, Table 5). Usually the segment length is difficult, if not impossible at times, to measure as it merges imperceptibly with the T wave. The segment, like J, is usually not shifted normally more than plus or minus 1 millimeter in the standard leads. Conditions which alter the position of J usually alter the position of the S–T segment. Myocardial infarction, pericarditis, trauma, cardiac hypertrophy or exercise in patients with coronary sclerosis are frequent etiologic factors responsible for displacement of the S–T segment. Segment displacements due to death of cardiac muscle or myocardial ischemia are usually *temporary,* whereas displacements due to cardiac hypertrophy or ventricular strain are usually *persistent.*

THE S–T INTERVAL

The duration of the S–T interval is a measure of the duration of the depolarized state plus that of repolarization. In most electrocardiograms there is no true isoelectric or S–T segment, because repolarization of some portions of the ventricle begins before or immediately after depolarization is completed. Furthermore, an isoelectric interval may also exist in the presence of repolarization electric forces if they fortuitously result in a net potential of zero. The duration of the S–T interval is not ordinarily employed clinically to determine the presence of cardiac disease. Instead the duration of the Q–T interval, which represents the time required for ventricular depolarization and repolarization, is employed. The configuration and position of the S–T segment and T wave, considered individually or collectively, have much clinical significance (*vide infra*).

THE T WAVE

The T wave, the wave of ventricular repolarization, is important in the electrocardiographic diagnosis of cardiac disease. It usually starts at the isoelectric line and rises gradually to its apex, descending to the isoelectric line somewhat more rapidly (Fig. 116).

The T wave may assume many shapes, some of which when present in certain leads under certain circumstances, indicate the presence of cardiac disease (Fig. 117).

The T waves are altered by many physiologic states other than those found in the presence of cardiac disease: (1) drinking of cold water just prior to an electrocardiographic examination; (2) therapeutic amounts of digitalis; (3) smoking; (4) extreme emotional upsets; and (5) variations in position of the heart. It is important to control these

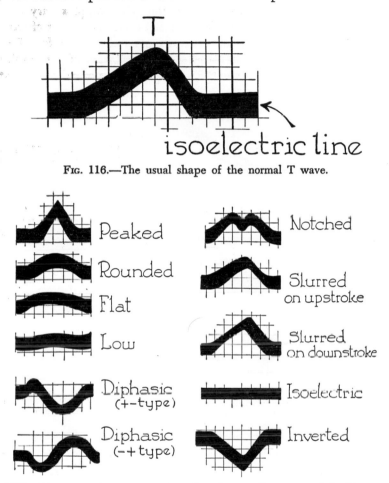

FIG. 116.—The usual shape of the normal T wave.

FIG. 117.—Diagrammatic representation of various configurations of the T wave seen in normal and diseased hearts.

factors when the significance of abnormal types of T waves are interpreted. The significance of such T wave changes often cannot be satisfactorily evaluated without measurement of the Ventricular Gradient (Chapter 5).

A negative T wave in lead I, for all practical purposes, is definite evidence of myocardial disease. Normally the T wave in this lead is usually greater than 0.5 millimeter. If the wave is smaller than this or if it is diphasic, the patient in all probability has cardiac disease. When the wave is deeply notched or deformed to a great extent, myocardial disease should be suspected. It may be said at this point that in general, when the QRS complex is large, the T wave following it tends to be large and when the QRS complex is small, the T wave tends to be small. Normally the T wave and the major deflection of the QRS complex vary concordantly. T wave (repolarization) changes that occur as a result of changes in the QRS complex (depolarization) are spoken of as *secondary T wave changes.* If the QRS complex in lead I is small, a T wave of low amplitude may not be abnormal. When the QRS complex is of normal configuration

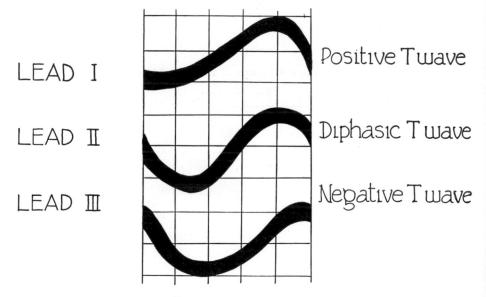

FIG 118.—Diagrammatic illustration of a diphasic T_2 produced by the algebraic addition of a positive T_1 and negative T_3.

and of normal size, and the T wave is abnormal, the change is spoken of as *a primary T wave change,* which is indicative of myocardial disease. It must be pointed out, however, that inversion of the T wave may be permanent or transient, depending upon the etiologic factors responsible for the change. If the cardiac disease is reversible, as for example anemic cardiac disease, the abnormal T wave is usually also reversible. If the cardiac disease is not reversible, as for example arteriosclerotic heart disease, the T wave usually remains inverted or abnormal.

In lead II a negative T wave is highly suggestive evidence of the presence of cardiac disease, as the T is seldom normally inverted in this lead if the subject is resting in the supine position during the recording of the electrocardiogram. A notched, isoelectric or diphasic T wave in lead II is not uncommon normally. Such waves are produced by the additive effects of normal T_1 and T_3 (Fig. 118).

The T wave in lead III is often inverted normally. In patients with a transverse heart, as in obese patients, the main deflection of the QRS complex in lead III is frequently negative and T_3 is also inverted (Fig. 119).

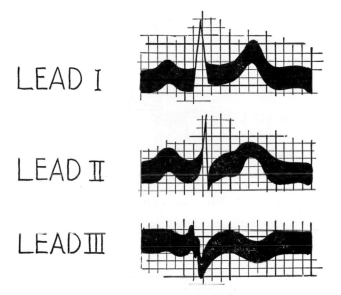

FIG. 119.—Inversion of the T wave in lead III in an *obese patient* with his heart in a transverse position.

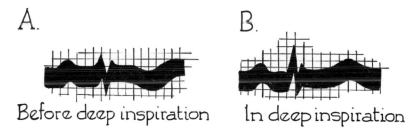

FIG. 120.—The effect of deep inspiration on an inverted T wave in lead III in a patient with a transverse heart.

With the descent of the diaphragm following deep inspiration, the heart becomes more vertical and the QRS complex and T wave often become positive (Fig. 120). In the normal heart, the negative T wave in lead III does not ordinarily exceed —3 mm.

Electric Axis of the T Wave.—The electric axis of the T wave is determined in the same manner as described for the QRS complex. It is necessary to measure the areas under the T waves for accurate determinations. The use of amplitude determinations will give only rough estimates of the electric axis of the T wave.

The electric axis of the T wave normally tends to follow that of the QRS complex, so that in patients with a transverse heart the deviation of the QRS to the left is associated with a deviation of the T wave to the left.

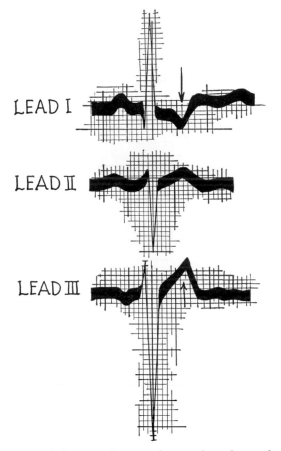

Fig. 121.—The main deflections of QRS and T are discordant in leads I and III.

The axis of the T wave tends to lie about 20 degrees to the left of the QRS axis. The electric axis of the T wave does not tend to follow rightward deviation of the QRS as closely. The direction of the T wave tends to follow the direction of the major deflection of the QRS complex, *i.e.*, the major deflection of the QRS and T wave are usually *concordant* (Figs. 119 and 120) normally.

When the direction of the T wave is opposite to the direction of the main deflection of the QRS complex, the T wave and QRS complex are said to be *discordant* (Fig. 121). This is usually associated with cardiac disease, especially that producing strain on the left ventricle. There results severe left axis deviation of the QRS, with right axis deviation of the T wave (Figs. 121 and 122).

The direction of the mean electric axis of the QRS complex (Fig. 121) is —50 degrees and that of the mean electric axis of the T wave is +117 degrees (Fig. 122).

As stated above, a negative T wave in lead II is strongly suggestive of myocardial disease only if the electrocardiogram has been taken with the *patient in the supine position.* Always record the electrocardiogram with

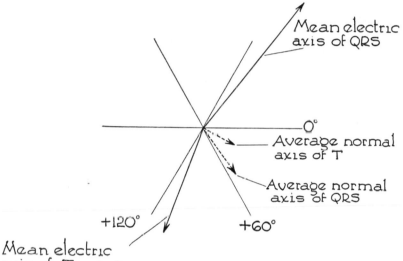

FIG. 122—A leftward deviation of the QRS and a rightward deviation of the T wave of the electrocardiogram of figure 121.

the patient in the same position, preferably the supine position, in order to control changes in T waves, QRS complexes and other portions of the electrocardiogram that may be influenced by a change in position of the subject from one recording to the next.

Abnormalities of the T waves can be produced by any type of cardiac disease and, in fact, by almost any disease state associated with toxemia which may injure the myocardium. Acidosis, insulin, carbon monoxide, hyperthyroidism and hypothyroidism, mitral stenosis, arteriosclerosis, nephritis, uremia, avitaminosis, hypertension, pneumonia, severe infections of any sort, and many other diseases and drugs have all produced changes in the T waves which were either transient or permanent. *In fact, any factor which can alter physicochemical biologic processes may alter the T wave, since the order of the repolarization process is extremely sensitive.*

8

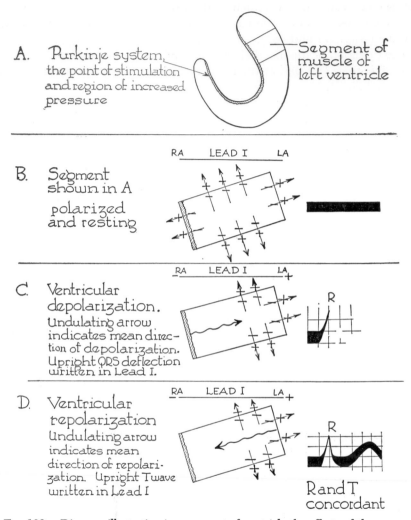

A. Purkinje system, the point of stimulation and region of increased pressure

Segment of muscle of left ventricle

B. Segment shown in A polarized and resting

C. Ventricular depolarization. Undulating arrow indicates mean direction of depolarization. Upright QRS deflection written in Lead I.

D. Ventricular repolarization Undulating arrow indicates mean direction of repolarization. Upright T wave written in Lead I

R and T concordant

Fig. 123.—Diagram illustrating in a segment of ventricle the effects of the processes of depolarization and repolarization upon lead I. The impulse reaches the subendo-cardial layer of muscle of the ventricle by way of the Purkinje system to initiate a depolarization process which migrates outward to the epicardial surface. This results in a negative potential in the cavity of the ventricle and a positive potential at the epicardial surface (part C). Repolarization begins at the epicardial surface and migrates inward to the endocardial surface, again resulting in a negative field in the cavity of the ventricle and a positive field on the epicardial surface (part D). The net effect is to produce concordant depolarization (R) and repolarization (T) waves. Similarly, in the auricle where the processes of depolarization and repolarization migrate parallel to the endocardial and epicardial surfaces and occur in the same order, the P wave and auricular T wave are discordant.

Generally speaking, *peaked T waves* may be seen in patients with tachycardia, regardless of etiology. Myxedema or hypothyroidism, obesity, edema, and pleural or pericardial effusions all produce low or *isoelectric T waves*. Such T wave changes are secondary to altered conductivity of the tissues except in hypothyroidism.

In the descriptions of the depolarization and repolarization processes of the hypothetic cell in Chapter 1, it was stated that the wave of the process of repolarization is opposite in direction to that of depolarization. In the human electrocardiogram the depolarization wave of the ventricles (QRS complex) and the repolarization wave of the ventricles (T wave) are usually and normally in the same direction, *i.e.*, concordant. The depolarization and repolarization waves of the auricles are in opposite directions, *i.e.*, discordant. The reasons for these differences are unknown, and any explanation is purely conjectural at this time, although it has been shown that pressure on a polarized tissue, if great enough, will retard repolarization. Therefore, the pressure in the auricles may not be sufficiently great to retard repolarization, so that the P and auricular T waves are normally discordant. On the other hand, the pressure inside the ventricle is high, and therefore repolarization in the endocardial region, where the pressure effect is greatest, is delayed so that the repolarization process starts at the epicardium and migrates toward the endocardium instead of migrating from the endocardium to the epicardium (Fig. 123). Whether or not the influence of pressure is the explanation for the normal discordant QRS and T waves is unknown.

In order to evaluate primary and secondary T wave changes properly, the use of the *ventricular gradient*, an expression of the variations in duration of the excited state in the ventricular musculature, is necessary. It is a method for expressing, localizing, and evaluating as a vector force the variations in duration of the excited state as it is influenced by both depolarization and repolarization processes. The gradient is discussed more completely in Chapter 5. Its study makes possible visualization of the relative directions and durations of the depolarization and repolarization processes.

DISEASE STATES THAT ALTER J, THE S–T SEGMENT AND THE T WAVE

Myocardial Infarction

For the purpose of this discussion, we shall consider infarction of the myocardium as occurring in one of three areas (see Chapters 3 and 4 for more detailed subdivisions):

1. Infarction of the *anterolateral and apical region of the left ventricle*, which is usually due to occlusion of the left coronary artery or the left anterior descending branch.

2. Infarction of the *basal posterior region of the left ventricle*, which is ordinarily due to occlusion of the right coronary artery or of the posterior descending branch of that artery.

3. Infarction of the *posterolateral regions of the left ventricle*, which is ordinarily due to occlusion of the circumflex branch of the left coronary artery (Fig. 124).

Anterolateral Myocardial Infarction.—Infarction of the myocardium as a result of occlusion of the left coronary artery or of the anterior descending branch of the left coronary artery that is strictly anterior results in no or few abnormalities *in the standard leads*. This is true because abnormalities occurring in the depolarization and repolarization processes

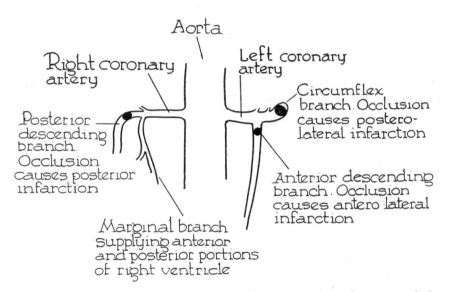

F₁G. 124.—A diagrammatic representation of the coronary arterial system and the common sites of coronary artery occlusion. Dark disks indicate sites of obstruction.

travel directly toward or away from the frontal plane of the body. Infarcts, however, are usually not strictly anterior. Generally, they involve the apical and septal portion of the left ventricle and the lateral wall and thus usually exert a visible electric effect on the three standard leads (Fig. 125). Changes in the behavior of the electric activity within the heart occur parallel to the frontal plane and influence the electrodes of the standard leads when the lateral surfaces of the heart are involved.

In *acute anterior infarction* the R wave in lead I becomes low and an abnormal Q wave appears. The S–T segment becomes extremely elevated and the T wave may disappear. In lead III the S–T segment becomes severely depressed and the T wave also may disappear (Fig. 126*B*). After a few hours or days the infarct begins to heal. The healing process (sub-

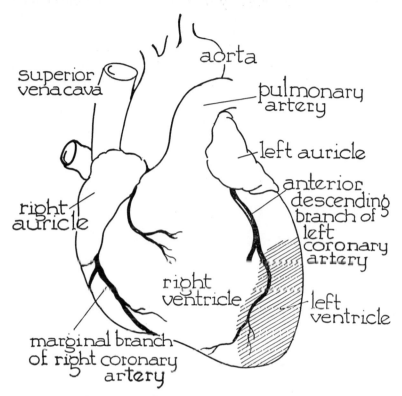

Fig. 125.—Common location for anterior myocardial infarct.

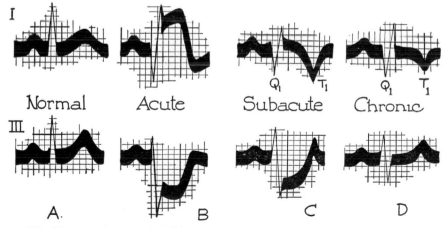

Fig. 126.—Diagrammatic representation of serial changes that occur in anterior myocardial infarction.

acute stage) is characterized by deepening of Q_1, return of the S–T_1 segment almost to the isoelectric line, and deepening of T_1. The S–T segment is smoothly curved or *coved*, producing the *Pardee type* of T wave (Fig. 126C). In lead III the S–T segment returns almost to the isoelectric line and the T wave becomes sharply upright. After a few weeks the infarct becomes *chronic* and is characterized by the presence of a Q_1 and

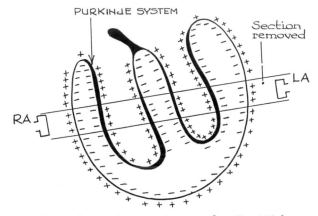

Fig. 127.—Resting human heart. A section is removed to Fig. 128 for careful analysis.

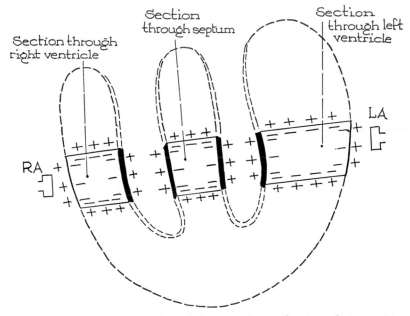

Fig. 128.—Transverse section through the entire heart, showing relative positions of the segments to each other and to the RA and LA electrodes of lead I. No difference in potential exists between the RA and LA electrodes when the heart is at rest and fully polarized.

often an inverted T_1, frequently called the Q_1T_1 pattern. After weeks, months or years T_1 may return to normal and in some cases the Q wave becomes very small or disappears, leaving no evidence of the previous infarct. Patients with large infarcts may retain the Q_1 for the rest of their lives.

Mechanism of Production of Electrocardiographic Pattern of Infarction.—In order to appreciate the electrocardiographic changes produced by infarction and to interpret tracings intelligently, one must understand the mechanisms involved. Although the discussion to follow concerns an anterolateral infarct and the Q_1T_1 pattern, the same explanation is applicable to any infarct, regardless of its location.

The normal resting heart is fully polarized, as shown in figure 127, and no difference in potential exists between the RA and LA electrodes of lead I. When an impulse is delivered to the subendocardial surface by the Purkinje system, a wave of depolarization migrates out perpendicular to the epicardium. After certain physicochemical processes have occurred the recovery process or wave of repolarization moves perpendicular to the endocardium, beginning at the epicardium.

For the sake of discussion, let us investigate a segment of muscle from the right and left ventricular walls and septum more carefully (Fig. 128). Before an impulse enters the Purkinje system from the AV node and bundle of His, it is first delivered to the subendocardial layer of muscle of the left side of the septum, and a wave of depolarization begins. Note that the wave is initiated in the left side of the septum, migrating toward the RA electrode and away from the LA electrode (Fig. 129A). This renders the RA electrode positive and the LA electrode negative; the galvanometer string therefore undergoes a negative or downward deflection and the downstroke of the *septal Q wave* is inscribed. Within 0.02 second or less the Purkinje system delivers the impulse to the subendocardial layer of muscle of the right and left ventricles and of the right side of the septum, thus inaugurating other waves of depolarization (Fig. 129B). Since the electric forces (*b* and *c*) due to the processes of depolarization from both sides of the septum are essentially equal and are acting in opposite directions, they cancel out. However, the muscular mass of the left ventricle is greater than that of the right ventricle, and the electric effects of depolarization in the left ventricle are directed more toward the left arm electrode than are the effects of the right ventricle toward the right arm electrode. In addition, the left arm is not as remote electrically from the left ventricle as is the right arm from the right ventricle. For this reason, the effective electric forces flowing toward the left arm electrode during depolarization of the ventricles is greater than that flowing toward the right arm, so that the left arm is rendered electrically positive and the right arm electrically negative. The galvanometer string moves to the positive side and the upstroke of the R wave is inscribed (Fig. 129B).

As the wave of depolarization continues through the walls of the heart, the potential differences decrease until, with completion of the process, there is no difference in potential; the galvanometer string then returns to the baseline, thus completing the downstroke of the R wave (Fig. 129C).

It is well to note that the direction of migration of the waves of depolarization is identical with the direction of flow of current in the heart. Remember that within the organism the current flows from the field of relative negativity to the field of relative positivity.

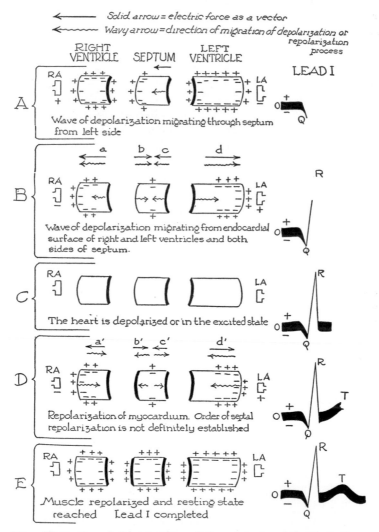

Fig. 129.—Illustration of the migration of the processes of depolarization and repolarization and their resultant forces in the normal heart. The influence of these forces on the RA and LA electrodes of lead I and the inscription of lead I are shown. See text for detailed description.

After certain physicochemical metabolic processes have occurred, a wave of repolarization begins. As noted previously, the process of recovery, regression, or repolarization begins where the process of excitation, accession or depolarization ended, *i.e.*, the waves of repolarization are initiated more or less simultaneously at the epicardial surfaces of the right and left ventricles and center of the septum (Fig. 129D). Because the electric (*b'* and *c'*) forces produced in the septum act in opposite directions, they cancel each other out. However, the electric force (*d'*) produced in the thick left ventricle is greater than that (*a'*) produced in the thinner right ventricular wall. The repolarization force in the left ventricle

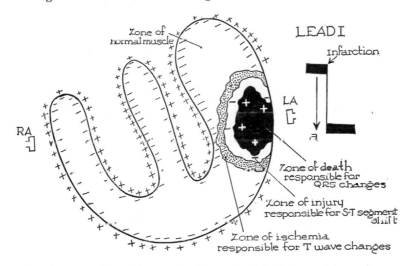

Fig. 130.—Diagram of an infarct in the free wall of the left ventricle, such as occurs in a strictly lateral or an anterolateral infarct. Consult the text for details.

is directed away from the RA toward the LA, whereas the smaller force in the right ventricle is in the opposite direction; the vector addition of the two forces (*a'* and *d'*) results in a vector force directed toward the LA, making the LA electrode positive and the RA electrode negative. Therefore, during the period of repolarization, the galvanometer string swings to the positive direction or upward in lead I, and a positive repolarization or T wave is inscribed (Fig. 129D). When the heart has been completely repolarized and the resting state has been achieved, no differences in potential will exist and the galvanometer string will swing back to the zero or isopotential line, completing the downstroke of the T wave (Fig. 129E).

Note that during the process of repolarization the direction of migration of the process and the resultant electric forces are conducted in opposite directions.

Zones in the Region of a Myocardial Infarct.—From a physiologic and electrocardiographic point of view the area of an infarct may be divided into the following zones (Fig. 130):

1. The *dead zone* is the central zone which is composed of dead cardiac muscle. This zone is free from any physiologic or active electrocardiographic phenomena and therefore may be considered a "physiologic hole or cavity" in the myocardium.

2. The *zone of injury* is a shell of cardiac muscle of variable thickness that surrounds the dead zone. The muscle in this zone is injured to a variable degree; some portions are progressing to recovery and others are regressing toward death. This zone is responsible for effects of *currents of injury* in the electrocardiogram.

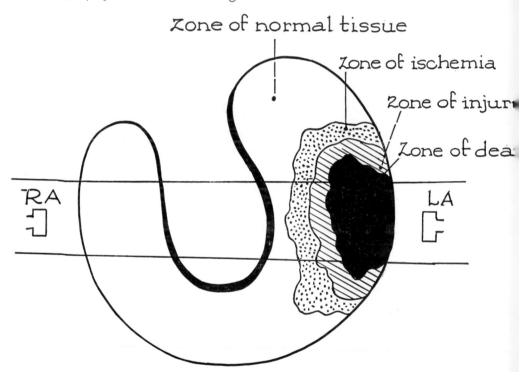

Zone of normal tissue

Zone of ischemia

Zone of injury

Zone of dead

RA

LA

Fig. 131.—Illustration of the transverse section of myocardium, transposed from the infarcted heart to figure 132 for detailed analysis. The septum is eliminated for convenience of illustration.

3. The *zone of ischemia* is a shell of cardiac muscle of variable thickness surrounding the zone of injury. The muscle in this zone is injured slightly, that is, to a lesser degree than the muscle of the aforementioned two zones. This zone accounts in particular for changes in the processes of repolarization reflected in the electrocardiogram as T wave changes.

4. The *zone of normal muscle* is the normal muscle enclosing the zone of ischemia.

It can be seen from figure 130 that the infarct has disturbed the state of polarization of the resting heart. In the dead zone the myocardium has become completely depolarized. With death of muscle or any cell, the gradient in ionic concentration is lost, so that potassium, sodium and other ions diffuse freely into and out of the dead cells until equal concentrations in the intra- and extracellular fluids result. Injured cells likewise have a reduction in the gradient in ionic concentration between the extra- and intracellular fluids, but since these cells are not killed, this gradient is not reduced to zero. Thus, the muscular cells in the injured zone behave as though they were in a medium of greater concentration of potassium along the outer surface with a loss of potassium from the interior. As a consequence, there is only partial depolarization of the shell of myocardium, which constitutes the zone of injury immediately surrounding the zone of dead myocardium (Figs. 130, 131 and 132). The effect is similar to that produced on the degree of polarization of the hypothetic cell. Potassium chloride was applied to half of its surface (Figs. 36 and 37, pages 41 and 42). Because the myocardial shell, which forms the zone of injury, is partially polarized and the subendocardial shell of normal muscle is fully polarized, the potential of the LA electrode is relatively negative and the RA electrode relatively positive (Figs. 130 and 132A). This potential difference causes the current to flow in the subject from the LA to the RA, and the galvanometer string is made to deflect in a negative direction or downward by this *"current of injury"* (u, Fig. 132A).

It is important to realize that in the recording of an electrocardiogram, when the shadow of the galvanometer string is brought to the center of the camera slit, all currents that tend to deflect the string away from the center are neutralized. These are essentially steady currents. If there is a current of injury, it is also neutralized by an equal amount of current from the circuit in the control box of the electrocardiograph (b, Fig. 132B). This phenomenon of neutralization is not encountered in ordinary, clinically recorded electrocardiograms.

If an impulse is delivered by the Purkinje system to the subendocardial layer of muscle of the right and left ventricles, a wave of depolarization is started in both ventricles and progresses towards the epicardium. The septum is omitted from the discussion and illustrations for convenience and also because its role is of little significance except in special situations. During the early phases of this process, the resulting electric force (a) produced in the wall of the right ventricle exceeds the magnitude of that (b) produced in the thin noninfarcted, subendocardial shell of muscle in the left ventricle. Therefore, the vector addition of forces a and b yields a force c, which is directed toward the RA electrode (Fig. 132C). The RA then is relatively positive and the LA is relatively negative. When such a polarity exists for lead I, the galvanometer string is deflected in the negative direction or downward, and the downstroke of a Q wave is inscribed (Fig. 132C). As the process of depolarization progresses, the right ventricle becomes completely depolarized while living muscle around the infarct in the thicker left ventricle is still being depolarized. This makes the LA electrode relatively positive terminally in the depolarization process with respect to the RA electrode and, therefore, the galvanometer string is deflected in a positive direction or upward. Because much of the left ventricle has been destroyed by the infarct, a relatively small R is produced as the terminal deflection of the QRS (Fig. 132D). The larger

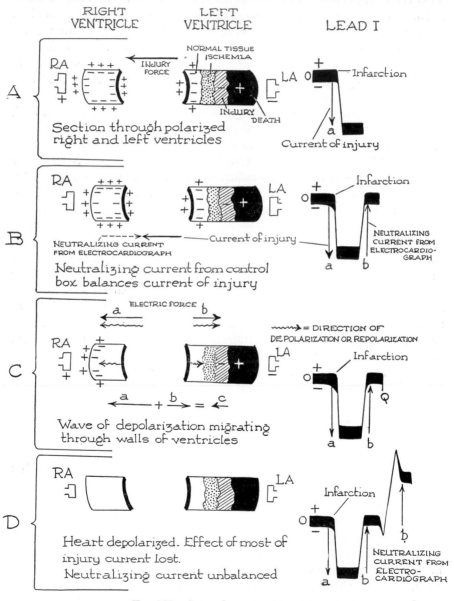

FIG. 132.—Legend on opposite page.

the infarct, the smaller will R_1 be. It is thus evident that *the dead zone or infarcted area itself is indirectly responsible for the Q_1 deflection and the small R wave or the QRS changes encountered in myocardial infarction. Therefore, without QRS changes a definite electrocardiographic diagnosis of infarction cannot be made.*

It can be seen in figure 132D that when the depolarization process is completed, the current of injury is almost completely, but not entirely, obliterated because in a living heart the muscle is not totally depolarized. With removal of the current of injury the neutralizing current from the electrocardiograph becomes unbalanced and therefore deflects the galvanometer string upward during the period when the heart is depolarized,

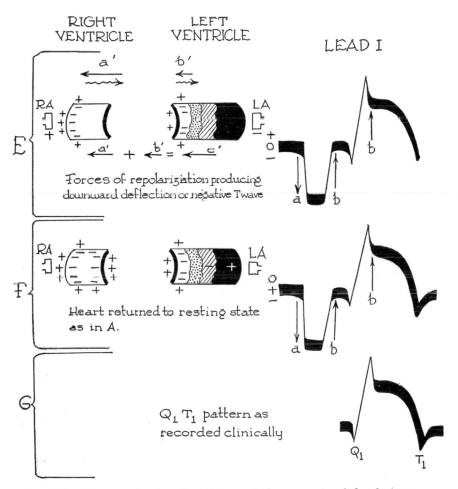

Fig. 132.—Diagram showing the influence of the processes of depolarization, repolarization, current of injury and neutralizing current from the electrocardiograph on the electrocardiogram in the case of an infarct involving the free wall of the left ventricle. Consult the text for details.

or when the S–T segment is being inscribed. This elevation of the S–T segment (Fig. 132D) is due indirectly to the current of injury but is directly attributable to the current from the control circuit of the electrocardiograph. It is thus evident that *a shift of the S–T segment is due to a current of injury or is due to the zone of injury.*

After a short time, during which physicochemical processes occur, the excited state begins to return to the resting state. The process of repolarization begins at the epicardial surface of the right ventricle and mi-

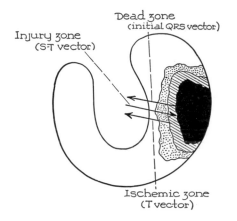

Dead zone
(initial QRS vector)

Injury zone
(S–T vector)

Ischemic zone
(T vector)

Fɪɢ. 133—It is evident from the text and from figure 132 that (1) the effective vector producing change in the initial portion of the QRS by the infarct is from the dead zone and can be represented by a vector extending from the centroid of the infarct to the centroid of the heart; (2) the effective vector producing change in the S–T segment by the zone of injury can be represented by a vector extending from the centroid of the heart to the centroid of the infarcted zone; (3) the effective vector produced by the zone of ischemia, which is responsible for the T wave change, may be represented by a vector extending from the centroid of the infarct to the centroid of the heart.

grates towards the endocardium. An electric force (a') is created that is directed toward the RA electrode. In the case of the infarcted region of the left ventricle, the area of ischemia retards the physicochemical processes concerned with recovery, just as they were delayed by cooling a surface of the hypothetic cell to 15° C. (Figs. 33 and 34). Therefore, repolarization begins at the subendocardial surface, where the muscle is more normal, and migrates toward the epicardial surface. The electric force (b') thus produced is directed toward the RA electrode. The vector sum of electric forces a' and b' results in force c' (Fig. 132E), which causes the RA to be relatively positive and the LA relatively negative. With such polarity of the arm potentials in lead I, the galvanometer string is directed downward (Fig. 132E). When the process of repolarization is complete, the galvanometer string returns to the zero or isopotential level

(Fig. 132E). Thus, it is evident that the *zone of ischemia is responsible for the T wave changes observed in infarction.*

Figure 133 shows that the electric force, which is due to the dead zone and is responsible for the changes produced in the initial portion of the QRS complex or depolarization wave, may be represented by a vector extending from the centroid of the infarcted zone to the centroid of the heart. The electric force responsible for the changes in the S–T segment, due to the zone of injury, may be symbolized by a vector electric quantity

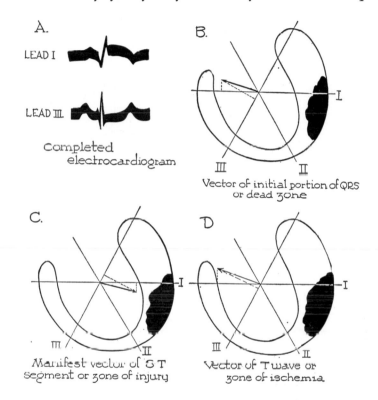

FIG. 134.—Diagram illustrating manner in which the three vectors shown in figure 133 can be used to predict the location of an infarct in the heart if the electrocardiogram is available, or how the electrocardiographic pattern may be predicted if the location of the infarct in the heart is known.

extending from the centroid of the heart to the centroid of the infarcted zone. The electric force responsible for the changes in the T wave, due to the zone of ischemia, may be denoted by a vector electric quantity extending from the centroid of the infarcted zone to the centroid of the heart.

Figure 134 shows the manner in which any or all of the three vectors, due to the zones of death, injury and ischemia, may be employed to predict the location of an infarct in the heart if the electrocardiogram is

available, or how the electrocardiographic pattern may be predicted if the
location of the infarct in the heart is known. The discussion of the unipolar precordial leads explains how an infarct may be located even more
precisely by taking advantage of these three vector forces (Chapter 3).

The same argument is applicable to any infarct, regardless of its location. Special consideration must be given to subendocardial infarction;
this should not be difficult if the infarct is placed subendocardially and the
same arguments are applied. This results in shifts "against the rule" for

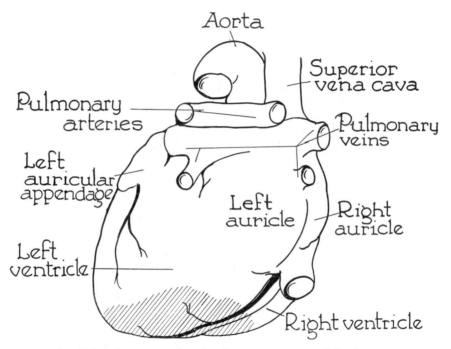

Fig. 135.—The common location for posterior myocardial infarction.

obvious reasons. Once the foregoing arguments for anterolateral infarction are comprehended, detailed explanation for each type of infarction
becomes unnecessary and will not be presented here.

Posterior Myocardial Infarction.—The area of infarction of the myocardium from occlusion of the right coronary artery or its main branch,
the posterior descending artery, includes the posterior portion of the
septum and diaphragmatic portion of the left ventricle (Fig. 135). In a
few subjects (about 10 per cent) the posterior portion of the left ventricle
is supplied by the left coronary artery.

If, in the pattern of the anterior infarct, leads I and III were inter-
changed, the electrocardiographic pattern of posterior infarction would
be obtained (Fig. 136). The S–T segment in lead III is elevated and the

S–T segment in lead I is depressed early. Q_3 tends to appear and R_3 to become small. If a Q_1 were present before the infarct developed, it would tend to disappear. As the infarcted area heals, Q_3 becomes more prominent, the S–T segments in leads I and II approach the isoelectric line, and T_3 becomes negative and T_1 sharply peaked, *i.e.*, a Q_3T_3 pattern develops with coving of the S–T segment in lead III, and a Pardee type of T wave in lead III develops. A Q_2T_2 pattern may also evolve. The infarct may finally heal after many weeks or years, with electrocardiographic changes comparable to those described for an anterior infarct.

The direction of the S–T segment shift in posterior myocardial infarction is indicated in figure 137. The arguments concerning the vector force involved follow the same line of reasoning as that presented for an anterior infarct.

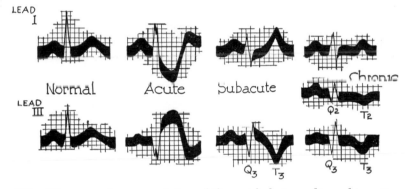

Fig. 136.—Diagrammatic representation of the serial electrocardiographic pattern of posterior myocardial infarction.

Posterolateral Infarction.—This usually results from occlusion of the circumflex branch of the left coronary artery. There may be no electrocardiographic manifestations in the standard leads in posterolateral infarction and, if present, they may last only a short time; thus, the condition is rarely diagnosed. Signs include depression of the S–T segment in leads I, II and 4V (Fig. 138). Use of multiple precordial leads usually localizes correctly the site of infarction (see Chapter 3). The T waves may be inverted. The condition often resembles effects of digitalis on the S–T segments and T waves. Since this type of infarct is more or less posterior, comparable to the strictly anterior infarct, there is usually little or no change in the QRS complex in the standard leads. The nature of the forces involved may be analyzed along the lines previously discussed for anterior and posterior infarction.

Infarcts may, of course, occur at any location in the heart, such as in the septum or in the auricles. They may be multiple, producing combined electrocardiographic pictures. They may occur at the endocardial or

9

epicardial surface and may be transmural or intramural. In the latter instance no effects of currents of injury are produced, as the forces about the infarcted area are equal and opposite in direction and balance each other (Fig. 139). If there are *multiple infarcts,* the electrocardiogram may

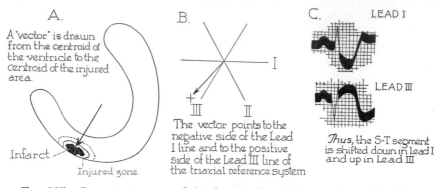

A. A "vector" is drawn from the centroid of the ventricle to the centroid of the injured area.

Infarct

Injured zone

B.

III   II   I

The vector points to the negative side of the Lead I line and to the positive side of the Lead III line of the triaxial reference system

C.   LEAD I

LEAD III

Thus, the S-T segment is shifted down in lead I and up in Lead III

Fig. 137.—In posterior myocardial infarction the S–T segment is shifted down in lead I and up in lead III. Consult figure 130 for electric activity of each zone in the region of the infarct. The "vector" indicated above is not a true vector, since its magnitude, as indicated, does not correctly represent the magnitude of the electric force involved. The magnitude may be found from the S–T segments of the electrocardiogram.

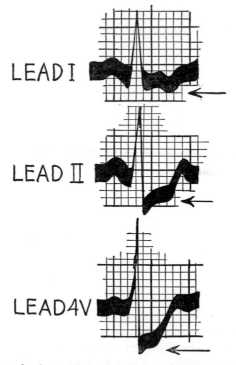

LEAD I

LEAD II

LEAD 4V

Fig. 138.—Posterolateral infarct. The arrows indicate depression of the S–T segments in leads I, II, and 4V. The QRS complexes remain more or less unchanged.

show some of the characteristics of all of them. The last one to develop and the largest usually predominate in the picture. Likewise, the infarct which, by virtue of its position, influences greatest the electrodes of the leads in use will tend to predominate in the finished record of those particular leads.

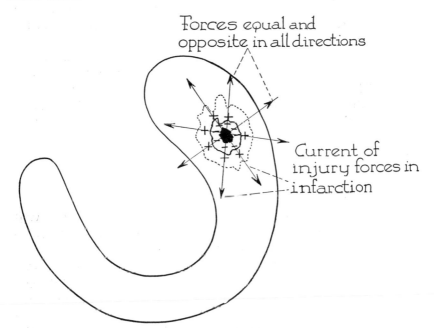

FIG. 139.—An *intramural* infarct produces no current of injury effects, as the forces produced are essentially equal and opposite in all directions. Since the injured zone behaves as though it were relatively negative, the polarization of the shell of injury will be shown in all similar figures to follow as in this figure.

Obviously, areas of the heart which are depolarized last or during the midtemporal period of ventricular depolarization cannot produce alterations in the process of depolarization early in the QRS complex. Thus, when these areas are depolarized, the mid or late portions of the QRS complex are changed. The changes are reflected by notches, slurs or other deformities. The changes are recognized much more readily by comparing serially recorded tracings. The tracings will not show Q waves as described above unless there is associated infarction of the areas of the heart which are depolarized early.

Pericarditis

The electrocardiographic signs of pericarditis are caused by inflammation of the subepicardial layer or shell of muscle. This condition is considered to be associated with a localized or generalized area of myocardial injury which, as in the case of myocardial infarction, produces a current of injury during the acute phase of the disease. The electrocardiogram usually manifests this type of myocardial injury but does not reveal its etiology. Rheumatic fever, tuberculosis, pyogenic infection, trauma, uremia, and other diseases may be etiologic agents. Pericarditis may be *acute, subacute,* or *chronic.* The acute form is seldom seen in patients with tuberculous pericarditis, as the onset is usually insidious. Furthermore, this disease does not remain acute long and the currents of injury are evanescent, so that electrocardiograms must be taken early and frequently to reveal the acute changes.

In *acute pericarditis,* usually any one of four electrocardiographic pictures is seen; however, less frequently, pictures other than these may be produced. The four characteristic patterns described in the clinical medical literature involve *elevations of the S–T* segment and depression or inversion of the T wave in any of the following leads or combinations of leads:

1. Lead I.
2. Lead I and lead II.
3. Lead I and lead 4V.
4. Lead I, lead II, and lead 4V.

If the picture is typical, the S–T segment is isoelectric in lead III. With the presence of localized areas of pericarditis in certain regions, however, the S–T segment in lead III may not be isoelectric.

It is better to remember that just as in the case of coronary occlusion, the direction of the S–T segment will depend upon the location of the area of the heart injured by the inflammatory process than it is to memorize the four patterns listed, which will not apply under all circumstances. In acute *diffuse* pericarditis, injury to the myocardium usually occurs so that there is a layer of injured muscle just under the epicardium surrounding the entire heart. By the same arguments as those presented in patients with myocardial infarction (Fig. 130), it is apparent that a "vector," drawn from the center (more correctly, the centroid) of the ventricles to the centroid of the injured area and analyzed on the triaxial reference system, will indicate the direction and lead or leads in which a shift of the S–T segment will take place (Fig. 140).

It can be seen that it is possible to have an elevation of the S–T segments in various combinations in the standard leads, and even to have a depression of the S–T segment in lead I or III, if the area of pericarditis is located in a particular place. There may be reciprocal shifting of the S–T segment in leads I and III in sharply localized areas of pericarditis. In fact, the S–T segment changes in such areas will be similar to those seen in the various types of myocardial infarction, if comparably placed. This is rather rare clinically, since pericarditis is usually diffuse, as the beating heart disseminates the infecting organisms throughout the pericardial sac almost immediately.

The electrocardiographic changes of *subacute pericarditis* are usually seen early, that is, within a matter of hours or days, as the inflammation or injury of the subepicardial muscle subsides quickly. At this time, with the return of the S–T segments toward the isoelectric line, the T waves decrease in magnitude and frequently become negative. The inversion of the T waves is usually not great. The T waves are frequently inverted in all standard leads and in lead V$_4$ (Fig. 141). In pericarditis there is a shell of myocardial ischemia which results in T wave changes. These changes, which may be analyzed on the triaxial reference system, result in a vector force originating in the centroid of the ischemic shell and directed toward the centroid of the heart.

In *chronic pericarditis* the electrocardiographic picture is usually not

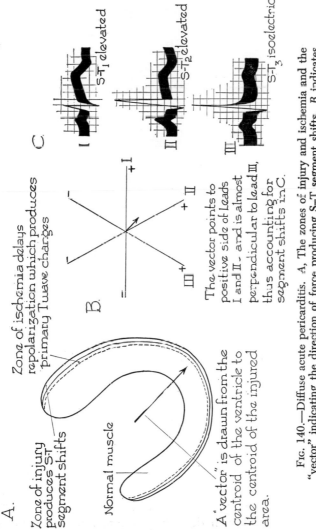

Fig. 140.—Diffuse acute pericarditis. A, The zones of injury and ischemia and the "vector" indicating the direction of force producing S–T segment shifts. B indicates the influence of the current of injury on the S–T segment in the three standard leads shown in C.

characteristic. In certain cases, however, the QRS complexes and the T waves are of low voltage, but the P waves are of normal or increased voltage. The QRS complexes may be splintered and the T waves may be low, flat, isoelectric or inverted in one or more of the standard leads (Fig. 142). Fixation of the heart in the thorax may sometimes be demonstrated

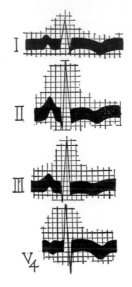

FIG. 141.—*Subacute pericarditis,* showing inverted T waves in leads I and II and in lead V₄. The S–T segments are essentially at the isoelectric line.

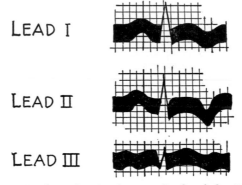

FIG. 142.—*Chronic pericarditis,* showing low amplitude of the QRS complexes and negative T waves with normal amplitude of the P waves.

in an electrocardiogram taken with the patient lying in the right lateral position, first in deep expiration, then in deep inspiration. If there is no change in the electric axis with this test, it suggests fixation of the heart, most likely by chronic adhesive pericarditis. In the normal subject the heart shifts to the right with deep inspiration, but in the presence of pulmonary disease, a large heart, or severe pericardial effusion, there may be fixation of the electric axis.

ANGINA PECTORIS

During the pain of angina pectoris, the electrocardiogram will show S–T segment and T wave changes—usually depression of all S–T segments and T waves in all leads, including the unipolar precordial leads (Fig. 143). When the attack of angina terminates, the electrocardiogram reverts to the preanginal pattern, since this is a reversible phenomenon.

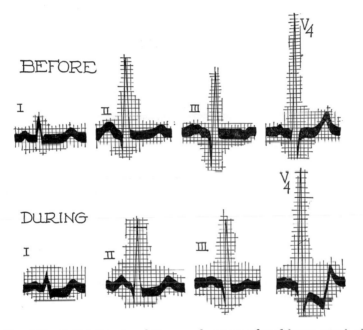

FIG. 143.—S–T segment and T wave changes produced by an attack of angina pectoris.

Characteristically, there are no QRS changes. One would not expect QRS changes physiologically, for if the pain is due to spasm followed by a temporary period of ischemia, only injury effects (temporary S–T segment shifts and T wave changes) would be expected. Since there is no death of muscle, QRS changes do not occur. The coronary spasm is only temporary, and therefore the S–T segment and T wave changes are transient also. Since the S–T segments of the precordial leads and standard leads are depressed, the injury must be subendocardial. In clinical practice, anginal pain is precipitated by exercise or by breathing gas low in oxygen, and an electrocardiogram taken prior to the attack should be compared with those obtained during and following the precipitated attack. Nitroglycerine will release the spasm and pain and will simultaneously restore the electrocardiogram to its preanginal characteristics.

Electrocardiographic differentiation of myocardial infarction, angina pectoris and pericarditis is not difficult. The pattern of the infarct, by definition, must have a zone of death. For the demonstration of such a zone electrocardiographically, there must be changes in the initial portion of

TABLE 1

Summary of electrocardiographic changes observed in myocardial infarction, angina pectoris and pericarditis which are of significance in their clinical electrocardiographic diagnostic differentiation.

ECG change	ZONE			Duration of ECG change
	Dead	*Injury*	*Ischemia*	
	Initial portion of QRS	*Shift of S–T segment*	*T wave*	
Myocardial infarction	Present	Present	Present	Hours to days to years
Angina pectoris	Absent	Present	Present	Only during attack
Pericarditis	Absent	Present	Present	Hours to days to years

the QRS complex, without which the electrocardiographic diagnosis can only be indirect. The final diagnosis is established on the basis of the entire clinical picture. Pericarditis and angina pectoris are assocated with S–T segment changes but not with QRS alterations. In the former the changes characteristically persist for hours, days or longer, whereas in the latter they last only for the duration of the anginal pain. Consult Table 1 for summary of the electrocardiographic diagnostic differentiation of these clinical states.

Left Ventricular Hypertrophy With and Without Ischemia
(Left Ventricular Strain)

It will be recalled that *left axis deviation* is characterized by an S_3, the amplitude of which is greater than R_3 and by an R_1 that is greater than R_2 or R_3. The conditions producing left axis deviation have already been discussed. In patients without serious myocardial disease and with left axis deviation, the S–T segments are usually isoelectric and the T waves are upright in leads I and II. The T waves in lead III are ordinarily low, isoelectric, or inverted (Fig. 144). With excessive "strain" on the left ventricle, as in patients with prolonged severe hypertension, the pattern of left ventricular "strain" develops (Fig. 144C). The S–T segment be-

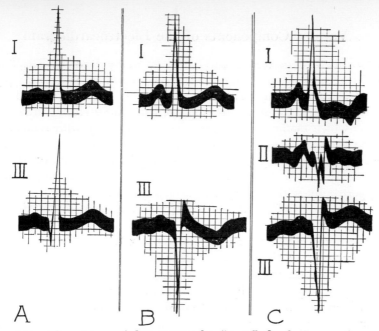

Fig. 144.—The picture of *left ventricular "strain"* developing as degenerative processes take place in the left ventricle. There is leftward deviation of the QRS complex, rightward deviation of the T waves and depression and elevation of the S-T segments in leads I and III, respectively. The T wave changes indicate anterolateral ischemia of the myocardium.

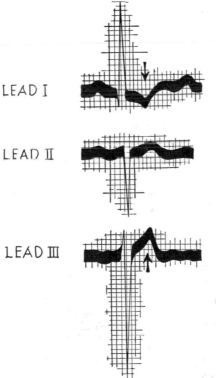

LEAD I

LEAD II

LEAD III

Fig. 145.—Extreme leftward deviation of the electric axis of the QRS and rightward deviation of the T wave in a patient with hypertension.

comes distinctly depressed in lead I and elevated in lead III. The T waves in lead I become sharply inverted and peaked and in lead III sharply upright and peaked. There is coving of the S–T segment in lead I. The term "left ventricular strain" is employed for those electrocardiographic patterns which manifest left ventricular hypertrophy with ischemia, *i.e.*, extreme left axis deviation with a late intrinsicoid deflection (see Fig. 200, page 194) and tendency to a wide QRS complex and T waves as described immediately above. In the absence of the T wave changes, there may be hypertrophy with the typical pattern. The term "strain pattern" is commonly employed but is not a desirable one from the electrocardiographic point of view.

The leftward deviation of the QRS complex is probably brought about by enlargement of the left ventricle and counterclockwise rotation of the heart about its longitudinal axis. The rightward deviation of the T waves is probably effected by ischemia* of the anterolateral portion of the myocardium, which alters and reverses the direction of the repolarization process. The hypertrophy itself or the increase in pressure in the interventricular cavity may be responsible for the alteration in order of repolarization. The S–T segment shifts, which are often greater than 1 millimeter, are difficult to explain. They may be brought about by currents of injury present in the left ventricle. Such a picture definitely indicates the presence of myocardial disease. Proger has stated that if there is extreme left axis deviation of the QRS and rightward deviation of the T wave, that is, if S_2 is more than 25 per cent of R_2 and T_3 is greater than T_1, then there is definite evidence of cardiac disease (Fig. 145). This is one way of describing severe leftward deviation of the mean electric axis of the QRS and rightward deviation of the axis of the T wave. These T wave changes are primary, *i.e.*, the order of repolarization is independent of the order of depolarization.

Acute Pulmonary Embolism

In *acute massive pulmonary embolism* the electrocardiographic pattern, in general, resembles posterior infarction with right axis deviation and is present only when acute embolism is associated with large areas of pulmonary infarction. The picture usually last only a few hours or days.

*The term ischemia is frequently loosely used in the field of electrocardiography. Unfortunately, it is too frequently considered to indicate inadequate blood supply. Although inadequate blood supply often produces alterations in the order of repolarization, metabolic disturbances of many sorts can produce changes in the S–T segment and T wave. It would seem desirable to modify its connotation to include disturbances in myocardial metabolism in which alterations in blood supply and ischemia can be one contributing factor. The general term, metabolic disturbances, would be more appropriate to define the physicochemical changes so often encountered in normal and abnormal physiologic disturbances which produce alterations in the S–T segment and T wave.

Serial electrocardiograms are useful in distinguishing this pattern from that of coronary occlusion; in embolism the electrocardiographic changes are transitory, whereas in infarction the alterations usually persist for weeks or months.

In pulmonary embolism there is characteristically a wide, large S wave in lead I. In leads II and III there are frequently Q waves and inversion of the T waves, although the former are not always present in lead II. The S–T segment is usually short or may often even be absent, so that

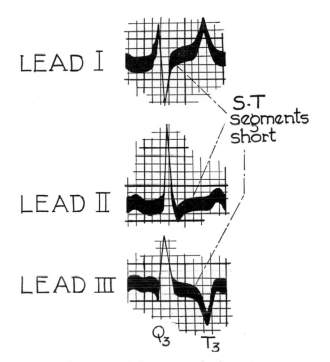

LEAD I

LEAD II

LEAD III

S·T segments short

Q_3 T_3

Fig. 146.—Acute pulmonary embolism. A wide, large S_1 is present with a Q_3T_3 pattern and shortening of the S–T segments. The duration of the QRS complex is greater than 0.10 sec.

the T wave comes directly from the QRS complex (Fig. 146). Lead III presents the Q_3T_3 pattern previously described for posterior infarction. Since the electrocardiographic picture is often incomplete, presenting only portions of the pattern described, serial electrocardiograms are helpful in suspected cases. In most instances of pulmonary embolism the electrocardiographic picture is not typical, although the changes are sufficient to indicate presence of the syndrome. The sudden strain on the right ventricle, with reflex coronary vasoconstriction, probably plays an important rôle in the production of the electrocardiographic syndrome.

Digitalis

Digitalis and allied drugs, in therapeutic amounts, usually produce changes limited to alterations in the S–T segment, J, and the T wave. Digitalis usually retards the cardiac rate and depresses the conducting system. As a result, there is prolongation of the P–R interval.

With *early digitalization* there is depression of the S–T segments in all limb leads if the main initial deflections of the QRS complexes are up in all leads. In general, the direction of the displacement of the segment is

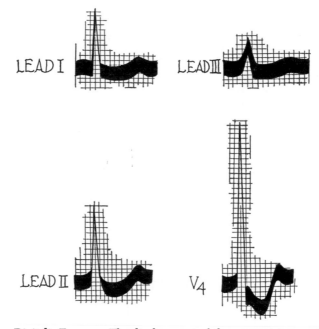

Fig. 147.—*Digitalis T waves.* The displacement of the segment is opposite in direction to the main deflection of the QRS complexes. J and S–T are depressed, and the T waves are diphasic of the minus-plus type.

opposite to the direction of the main initial QRS deflection (Fig. 147). Thus, if the patient has left axis deviation, there is a depression in lead I and an elevation in lead III. In lead V_4 the displacement is down. The S–T segment is not coved by digitalis, but essentially a straight line (Fig. 147).

With *more intensive digitalization,* J becomes shifted in the same direction as the S–T segment. In the normal standard leads and in lead V_4 the T waves become diphasic of the minus-plus type, so that most of the wave is below the isoelectric line. At this stage full digitalization is usually present.

With *overdigitalization,* multiple, multifocal premature beats, and coupling, auricular fibrillation or flutter, paroxysmal atrial tachycardia with blocks, and/or variable degrees of AV block may be produced.

Approximately three weeks are required after cessation of digitalis therapy for the electrocardiographic effects to disappear.

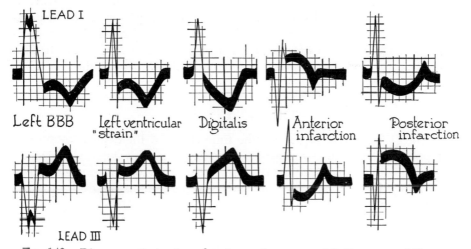

Fig. 148.—Diagrammatic tracings showing various types of S–T segment shifts and T waves.

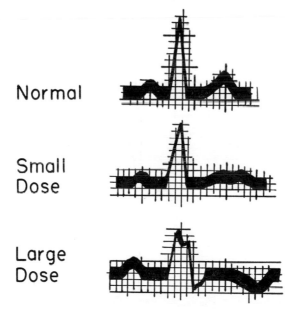

Lead I

Fig. 149.—Changes in the P wave, QRS complex and T wave produced by increasing doses of quinidine.

QUINIDINE

Quinidine and related drugs in therapeutic amounts tend to depress the electrical activity of the heart. The P wave is increased in duration with a slight increase in amplitude. The QRS duration is also increased and there is a tendency for a wide S wave to develop. The T wave is lowered, notched and widened. The Q–T interval is increased in duration because of depression of the depolarization and repolarization processes (Fig. 149). In toxic amounts, irregularities in cardiac mechanism and varying degrees of depression of conduction in the conduction tissue and myocardium develop.

THE Q–T INTERVAL

The *Q–T interval* represents the time required for depolarization and repolarization of the ventricular musculature. This interval coincides closely with mechanical ventricular systole, as systole begins essentially with the peak of the R wave and ends near the termination of the T wave. The interval is measured from the beginning of the QRS complex to the end of the T wave (see Chapter 1). It varies considerably with age, sex, and cardiac rate. When the rate is rapid, the interval is short and vice versa. The upper limits of normal for the duration of the Q–T interval at cardiac rates of 70 or greater is 0.42 second for women and 0.41 second

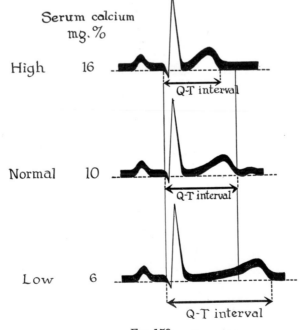

FIG. 150.

for men and children. The upper limits of normal are shown in detail in the Appendix, Table 8.[17] This table should be consulted in individual cases. Certain formulae are available for calculating the normal Q–T interval. The one presented by Ashman may be used:

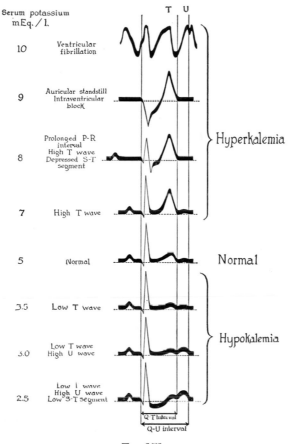

FIG. 151.

$$Q\text{–}T = K \log [10 (c + k)].$$

        k is a constant equal to 0.07 second.

        For women 15–35 years of age,

            K = 0.385 second

        For young men and for children in early infancy,

            K = 0.375 second

        For subjects 45 years of age and older,

            K = 0.380 second for men and 0.390 for women.

The Q–T interval *varies inversely with the calcium level of the blood.* When the concentration of calcium is high, the Q–T interval becomes shortened, and when it is low, the interval lengthens (Fig. 150). During

these changes the configuration of the T wave remains essentially un-
altered, that is, the ascending limb of the T wave rises slowly and the
descending limb declines more rapidly. In hypoparathyroidism or uremia,
after vomiting or forced breathing, or in cases of low calcium blood level,
the interval is prolonged. In hyperparathyroidism, if the blood calcium

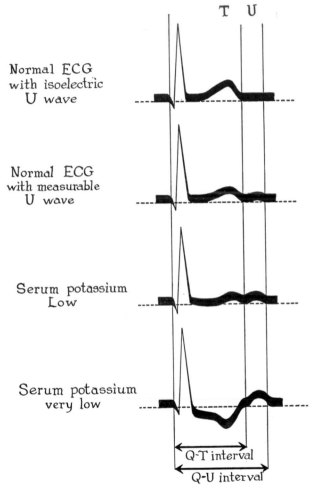

FIG. 152.

level is high, the interval is shortened. Digitalis will also shorten the
interval. Toxic states, myocardial ischemia, and various types of cardiac
disease, such as rheumatic, diphtheritic, arteriosclerotic, and hypertensive,
prolong the interval. A prolonged Q–T interval frequently indicates the
presence of myocardial disease. The return of the Q–T interval to normal
depends upon the reversibility of the disease. Hypopotassemia or hypokalemia depresses the S–T segment, lowers the T wave, increases the magni-

tude of the U wave, and causes the T and U waves to fuse (Fig. 151). These combined changes render the Q–U interval measurable. When the heart rate is taken into consideration, the Q–T interval as such is not actually increased, nor is the Q–U interval (Fig. 152). Hyperkalemia first causes the T wave to increase in magnitude, the S–T segment to become depressed, the U wave to disappear, and the QRS complex to increase in duration (Fig. 151). With further elevation of concentration of potassium in the serum and disturbance in potassium metabolism, the P–R interval is increased, the configuration of the P wave is changed, its magnitude is decreased, and it tends to migrate into the terminal portion of the preceding T wave, where at times it may be lost, even though auricular contractions continue (Fig. 151). As the potassium level rises, the duration of the QRS complex increases to produce patterns of complete bundle branch block (Fig. 151). Ventricular fibrillation may develop finally. Administration of rubidium and cesium tend to produce changes similar to those of potassium. Unfortunately, the underlying cardiac disease, with its associated electrocardiographic abnormalities, modifies the aforementioned patterns. Furthermore, a pure or single electrolyte disturbance is rarely encountered in man, and disturbances in the other electrolytes, including concentration of the hydrogen ion, can change the electrocardiogram in such a way as to simulate especially the patterns of hypokalemia. Because of these similarities, it is often possible to know only that disturbances in electrolytes exist, the nature of the disturbance being determined by other clinical and laboratory data. The electrocardiogram cannot be employed reliably or without extreme caution to indicate the concentration of potassium in the serum.

THE U WAVE

The U wave represents the positive after-potential and the period of greatest excitability of the ventricles. It tends to be of greatest magnitude in V_3. It is always positive normally in the standard limb and precordial leads and is usually in the same direction as the T wave but may be negative normally in Leads III, V_R, and V_F and the precordial leads when the T waves are negative. Ventricular hypertrophy, bradycardia, hyperthyroidism, hypokalemia, digitalis, epinephrine and hypercalcemia tend to increase the magnitude of the positive U wave. Hyperkalemia and other disturbances in electrolyte and acid-base balance may be associated with inverted U waves. Disease states of the myocardium that invert the T wave in any given lead may, but do not necessarily, invert the accompanying U wave. As with the T wave, the U wave may be diphasic or otherwise modified in configuration. The fact that the U wave is not always clearly discernible in conventionally recorded electrocardiograms reduces its usefulness in the interpretation of electrocardiograms.

10

Chapter 3

PRECORDIAL LEADS

An understanding of the precordial leads is not difficult if the nomenclature and method of recording the various leads and the depolarization processes presented previously are fully understood.

Precordial leads were the first leads used in electrocardiography. Ludwig and Waller, in 1887, used precordial leads when experimenting with a fairly insensitive capillary electroscope. When Einthoven brought forth his sensitive string galvanometer, little attention was paid to the use of precordial leads. In 1932 Wolferth and Wood published the first clinical paper on the use of these leads. Prior to this time, others, including Sir Thomas Lewis and Dr. F. N. Wilson and their associates, had published experimental studies with the use of precordial electrodes, but they had not organized the use of these leads for the clinician. The precordial leads of Wolferth and Wood and others, until 1938, were usually recorded upside down, as the electrodes were so connected that when the precordial electrode was relatively positive, a downward deflection resulted in the finished record and, when negative, an upward deflection was written. In 1938 the method of taking the precordial leads was standardized by a Committee representing the American Heart Association and the Heart Association of Great Britain and Ireland. Connections are now made so that *when the precordial electrode is relatively positive*, an upright wave is inscribed, and *when it is relatively negative*, a downward deflection is inscribed. This Committee also defined each type of precordial or chest lead as described hereafter.

The terms *fourth leads, chest leads* and *precordial leads* are used interchangeably and are, for practical clinical purposes, synonymous.

When chest leads are taken, two electrodes are used. The electrode placed over the region of the heart is called the *exploring, chest, or precordial electrode*. The other electrode, which is placed at a distance from the heart, is called the *indifferent electrode*.

Any one of the three standard leads may be converted into precordial leads in the following manner: One electrode of any lead which, when relatively positive, produces an upward deflection of the string is placed on the chest as the exploring electrode, and the other electrode of the same lead is placed at a distant fixed point on the body so that it will be influenced relatively little by the electric activity of the heart. The tracing is made with the electrocardiograph connected to the lead formed by the two electrodes. For example, it was stated that in the standard leads

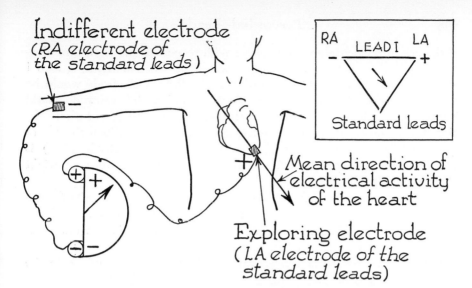

FIG. 153.—Lead I used as a precordial lead. When the precordial electrode is relatively positive, an upward deflection is inscribed.

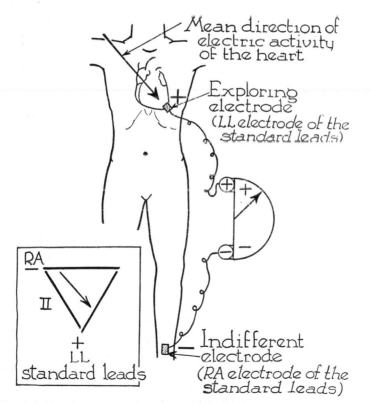

FIG. 154.—Lead II used as a precordial lead. When the precordial electrode is relatively positive, an upward deflection is inscribed.

if the left arm electrode were positive with respect to the right arm electrode in lead I, an upright deflection would be written. Thus, if lead I were used for recording the precordial leads, the LA electrode would be placed on the chest as the *exploring electrode* and the RA electrode would be placed at a distant fixed point on the body as the *indifferent electrode,* the galvanometer would be set for a lead I recording. When the forces produced by the heart are such that the exploring electrode (LA) is relatively positive and the RA electrode relatively negative, an upright deflection will be written.

In the average normal heart the electric activity travels in the frontal plane in the general direction running from the shoulders toward the pubis and legs and from right to left, that is, essentially from right shoulder to left iliac crest (Fig. 153).

If lead II were used as a precordial lead, the electrode, which in the standard leads is ordinarily placed on the left leg—the *LL electrode*—would be placed over the heart as the *exploring electrode.* The electrocardiograph is so constructed that when this electrode is relatively positive, a positive or upward deflection would be written. The other electrode of lead II of the standard leads, the *RA electrode,* is attached to a distant point on the body, usually the left leg, to form the *indifferent electrode.* The electrocardiogram is recorded with the electrocardiograph set for lead II. When the electric activity of the heart travels from the endocardium of the ventricles to the epicardium, the nearby precordial electrode will be more positive than the indifferent distant electrode, and an upward deflection of the string results (Fig. 154). When the polarity is reversed, the deflection is down.

One may use lead III as a precordial lead by connecting the *LL electrode* of the standard leads to the precordium as the *exploring electrode* and the LA electrode of the standard leads to the left leg as the *indifferent electrode* and then recording the electrocardiogram with the electrocardiograph set for a lead III recording. These are the connections usually made for ordinary clinical purposes.

It is well to note, however, that the indifferent electrode is not electrically remote enough from the heart to be uninfluenced by the electric cardiac activity; therefore, the completed electrocardiogram recorded with the exploring electrode over the precordium and the indifferent electrode at some remote point on the body represents a mechanical algebraic summation of the potential variations at these two electrodes. Such a recording is bipolar, just as are the standard leads. It is true that in many clinical circumstances the influence of the potential variations at the point of the indifferent electrode may not have much clinical significance, but the number of instances in which it is important is sufficiently great to warrant the recommendation that bipolar precordial leads be omitted except for special experimental purposes. For clinical as well as experimental purposes, the unipolar leads alone should be employed for exploration of the heart. In fact, only unipolar leads can be used for routine recording of the limb potentials. For this reason, unipolar limb leads and precordial leads are discussed in detail in this monograph. The bipolar leads are mentioned for precordial study only to the extent considered necessary for orientation. These will most likely be eliminated from clinical electrocardiography within the next few years by most individuals seriously interested in this subject.

SINGLE PRECORDIAL LEADS

The single precordial leads employed today are the 4F, 4R, 4L, 4B and 4V leads. These are sometimes written with the Roman rather than the Arabic numeral, for example IVF, IVR. The *numeral indicates the posi-*

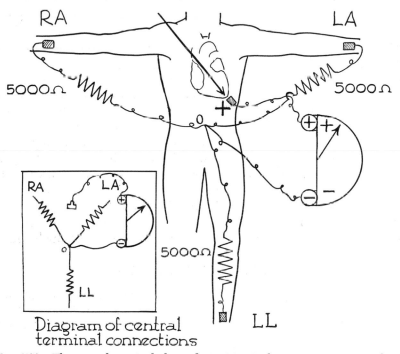

Diagram of central terminal connections

FIG. 155.—The central terminal electrode position is the most accurate one for the indifferent electrode for recording precordial leads. When the exploring electrode is relatively positive with respect to the other connections, an upright or positive deflection is written.

tion of the exploring electrode and the letter the position of the indifferent electrode. The numeral 4, or IV, indicates that the *precordial or exploring electrode* is placed over the apex of the heart *regardless* of its position. If the patient has dextrocardia, the electrode is placed over the right side of the chest over the apex or slightly lateral to it. If the apex cannot be located precisely by ordinary methods of physical examination, then it must be located fluoroscopically. It is necessary that the exploring electrode be placed precisely in order to avoid any serious errors. The *letter indicates the position of the indifferent electrode,* which is usually placed in the following locations, depending upon the lead desired:

F (Foot, *i.e.,* on the left leg just above the ankle)

R (Right arm, *i.e.,* on the right forearm just above the wrist)

L (Left arm, *i.e.,* on the left forearm just above the wrist)

B (Back, *i.e.,* at the inferior angle of the left scapula)

V (a central terminal formed by connecting the RA, LA, and LL electrodes to form the indifferent lead. See Fig. 155).

The 4V, which is a central terminal lead, is made by using as the indifferent electrode a central terminal formed by connecting the RA, LA, and LL electrodes. This indifferent electrode is connected to the negative pole of the galvanometer. The other pole of the galvanometer terminates in the *exploring electrode* (Fig. 155).

The central terminal lead is the most accurate method for recording the precordial leads, although *lead 4F is frequently employed clinically.* The former is more accurate, because the central terminal, for all practical purposes, is isopotential at all times during the cardiac cycle. The slight changes in potential which occur at the central terminal during the cardiac cycle are of little significance clinically. These slight changes are attributable to the fact that the heart is eccentrically located in the chest (anteriorly placed), and the three limbs are not equally remote electrically. In the other types of leads (4F, 4R, 4B, etc.) it is obvious that the *indifferent electrode* on the left leg, arm or back is not truly isopotential or *indifferent* during the entire cardiac cycle, as the electric activity from the heart exerts some influence on the distant electrode as well as upon the exploring electrode which is near the heart.

UNIPOLAR LIMB LEADS

F. N. Wilson and his associates, as well as others more recently, have employed unipolar limb leads in order to determine the electric potential at each of the three limbs; right arm (V_R), left arm (V_L) and left leg (V_F). In order to record the limb potentials, the connections are made as described for central terminal (V) leads. Three separate recordings are made serially with the precordial electrode placed near the right wrist (V_R), then near the left wrist (V_L) and then near the left ankle (V_F). Since the indifferent electrode placed at the central terminal is essentially isopotential at all times, the completed record indicates the variations in electric potential at each limb during each cardiac cycle. E. Goldberger has introduced the "augmented unipolar extremity leads" (aV) in order to increase the amplitude of the recorded limb potentials. To make such recordings, it is necessary to interrupt the connection to the central terminal from the extremity upon which the exploring electrode is placed. The completed augmented unipolar leads are known as aVr, aVl, and aVf leads, respectively.

V_R, V_L and V_F are, of course, directly related to the standard leads. Any two leads of these two sets furnish all the data necessary for calculating the deflection of the other four. It is not possible to enter into a mathematical discussion of the manner in which the three unipolar limb leads and the precordial leads might be used to calculate the potentials of the standard leads or vice versa. The following equations may be employed for such calculations:

$$V_F = \frac{e_2 + e_3}{3}$$

$$V_R = -\frac{e_1 + e_2}{3}$$

$$V_L = \frac{e_1 - e_3}{3}$$

$$-V_4 = e_4 - \frac{e_2 + e_3}{3},$$

where e_1, e_2, and e_3 are the potentials of each standard lead.

Furthermore, Einthoven's law states that the magnitude of any complex in lead I plus the complex recorded simultaneously in lead III is equal to the complex in lead II, or

Lead I + lead III = lead II, or
$(V_L - V_R) + (V_F - V_L) = V_F - V_R$, or
$V_F - V_R = V_F - V_R$.

It is also obvious that the sum of the magnitudes of the potentials of any complex recorded simultaneously for V_R, V_L, and V_F is equal to zero.

These leads have many applications in health and disease. They are particularly useful in detecting the electric position of the heart. The configuration of the complexes in the completed record is determined largely by the spatial position of the heart in relation to the three limb lead positions. Since the right shoulder and, in turn, the right arm, are directed into the atrioventricular orifices and cavities of the ventricles, a negative deflection is recorded for V_R. The relative spatial positions of the two ventricles, their muscular masses and orders of depolarization and repolarization influence the configurations of the complexes in V_L and V_F. In the normal subject with a horizontal heart the large mass of muscle of the left ventricle is directed toward the left arm. Because of the greater electric effects in a direction from endocardial surface to epicardial surface in the left ventricle than in the right ventricle, there results a great

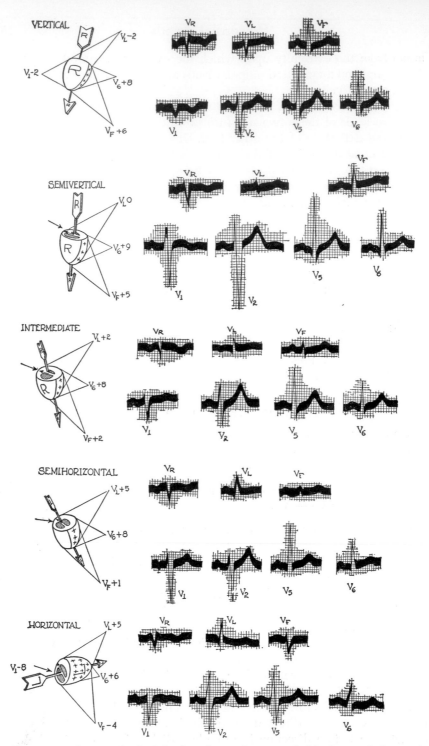

Fig. 156.—The unipolar limb leads and unipolar precordial leads recorded over the right (V₁ and V₂) and left (V₅ and V₆) sides of the heart, illustrating the various *electrocardiographic positions* of the heart. Although a general relation to anatomic

positive potential at the left shoulder or left arm during most of the period of ventricular depolarization. V_L, therefore, has a form similar to V_5 and V_6, *i.e.*, the QRS complex is mainly upright. For similar reasons, V_F has a form similar to V_1 and V_2, *i.e.*, the QRS complex is mainly down. In a vertical heart, the heart is rotated clockwise about its longitudinal anatomic axis and the left ventricle is directed toward the left leg. V_F, therefore, is similar to V_5 and V_6, and V_L is similar to V_1 and V_2. The criteria listed below, taken from Wilson and his associates, indicate electrocardiographically various positions of the normal heart. From the theoretic discussions presented elsewhere, it is possible to predict and understand the changes in the unipolar limb leads in infarction, bundle branch block, ventricular premature contractions, and other conditions. A detailed analysis of these special problems would not be suitable here.

The configurations of the deflections in the unipolar limb leads for six electrocardiographic positions of the heart are (Fig. 156):

Vertical Position.

(a) The ventricular complexes of lead V_L resemble those of leads V_1 and V_2.

(b) The ventricular complexes of lead V_F resemble those of leads V_5 and V_6.

---

position is shown in these illustrations, the electrocardiographic position and the anatomic position may vary independently. Some discrepancies are evident from these illustrations.

In the *vertical position*, the QRS complex of lead V_L resembles those of leads V_1 and V_2, and the QRS complex of lead V_F resembles those of leads V_5 and V_6, mainly because the large mass of muscle which forms the free wall of the left ventricle is directed away from the L electrode and toward the F electrode. The muscular mass of the left ventricle is so directed because of rotation of the heart to the right about the anterior-posterior axis and clockwise rotation about the anatomic axis. The large arrow through the longitudinal axis of the heart and the arrow in the septum are shown to aid in visualizing the rotations in all diagrams shown. The letters on the head and tail of the arrow indicate extent and direction of longitudinal rotation. The relationship of the arrow in the septum to that outside the heart, directed perpendicular to the base, also shows extent and direction of clockwise and counterclockwise rotation. When these two arrow heads point directly toward each other, the position about the longitudinal axis is intermediate. The large arrow through the longitudinal axis of the heart aids in visualizing rotation about the anterior-posterior axis.

In the *semivertical position*, the QRS complexes of lead V_F resemble those of leads V_5 and V_6, and the QRS complex of V_L is low in amplitude.

In the *intermediate position*, the QRS complexes of V_L and V_F are similar in form and size and resemble those of V_5 and V_6.

In the *semihorizontal position*, the QRS complex of lead V_L resembles those of V_5 and V_6, and the QRS complex of V_F is small.

In the *horizontal position*, the QRS complex of V_L resembles those of V_5 and V_6, and the QRS complex of V_F resembles those of V_1 and V_2. The discrepancy between V_F and V_2 and between V_L and V_5 is due to the extreme counterclockwise rotation about the longitudinal axis of the heart. Such discrepancies due to rotation about the longitudinal axis are rather common.

Semivertical Positions.

(a) The ventricular complexes of lead V_F resemble those of leads V_5 and V_6.

(b) The QRS deflections of lead V_L are small.

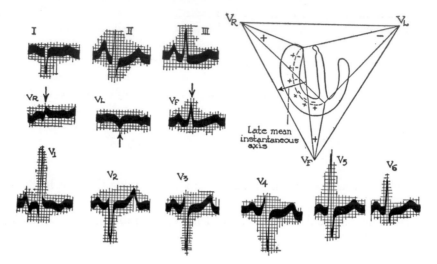

FIG. 157.—The unipolar limb leads in right ventricular hypertrophy with right axis deviation. V_R is mainly positive, V_L negative, and V_F positive. The arrows shown in association with the unipolar limb leads indicate that the thick right ventricular wall results in a late deflection.

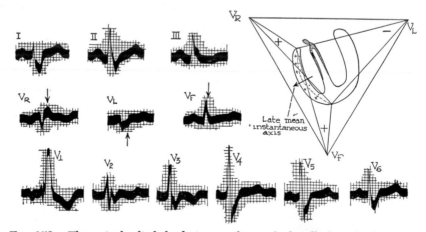

FIG. 158.—The unipolar limb leads in complete right bundle branch block. The arrows shown in association with V_R, V_L, and V_F indicate the deformed late portion of the QRS complex, which is the result of the late invasion of the right ventricular musculature and disturbed order of depolarization. The main deflection (one of longest duration and most deformed) is positive in V_R and negative in V_L.

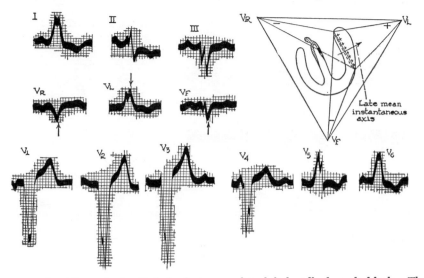

Fig. 159.—The unipolar limb leads in complete left bundle branch block. The arrows shown in association with V_R, V_L, and V_F indicate the deformed late portions of the QRS complex, which are the result of the late invasion of the left ventricular musculature and disturbed order of depolarization. The main deflection (one of longest duration and most deformed) is negative in V_R and positive in V_L.

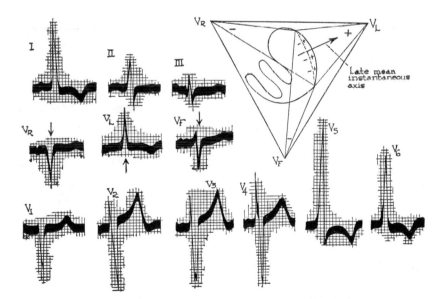

Fig. 160.—The unipolar limb leads in left ventricular hypertrophy. The arrows shown in association with V_R, V_L and V_F indicate the influence of the left ventricular hypertrophy on the magnitude, direction and duration of the QRS complexes in these leads. The QRS complex is large in amplitude and negative in V_R and is positive in V_L.

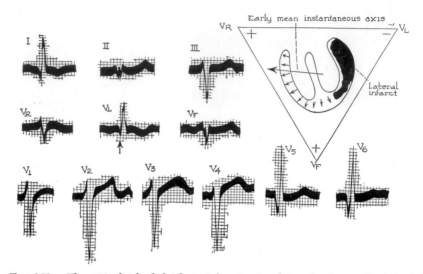

FIG. 161.—The unipolar limb leads in infarction involving the free wall of the left ventricle. The electrocardiographic pattern of infarction is shown in V_L, as well as in lead I and in V_5 and V_6. The arrow in association with V_L indicates the change in the initial portion of the QRS complexes (Q wave inscribed) produced by the infarction.

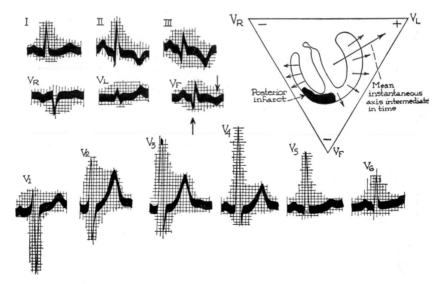

FIG. 162.—The unipolar limb leads in infarction involving the diaphragmatic (posterior-inferior) surface of the heart. The electrocardiographic pattern of infarction is shown in V_F and lead III. The Q wave indicated by the arrow represents the change in the initial portion of the QRS complex produced by the infarct.

Intermediate Postition.

(a) The ventricular complexes of leads V_L and V_F are similar in form and size and like those of leads V_5 and V_6.

Semihorizontal Position.

(a) The ventricular complexes of lead V_L resemble those of leads V_5 and V_6.

(b) The QRS deflections of lead V_F are small.

Horizontal Position.

(a) The ventricular complexes of lead V_L resemble those of leads V_5 and V_6.

(b) The ventricular complexes of lead V_F resemble those of leads V_1 and V_2.

Indeterminate Position.

There is no obvious relationship between the ventricular complexes of the limb leads and those of the precordial leads.

Figures 157 through 162 show variations in the unipolar leads in several clinical states. With ischemia of the lateral wall, the T waves in V_L tend to be reduced in magnitude or depressed. Similar changes may be produced by cardiac position. With infarction of the lateral wall of the left ventricle, the Q–T pattern as described for lead I also develops in V_L (Fig. 161). This pattern is likely to be especially helpful in clinical diagnosis when the pattern in lead I is not typical, such as in high lateral infarcts. On the other hand, the Q–T pattern of myocardial infarction of the diaphragmatic surface of the heart develops in lead V_F (Fig. 162). Unfortunately, just as with the Q_3T_3 pattern in lead III, the position of the heart and other cardiac and extracardiac factors make the pattern in V_F somewhat unreliable unless absolutely typical.

Right Ventricular Hypertrophy

When the right ventricle becomes hypertrophied and thick with a greater than normal mass of muscle it tends to have a predominating influence over the left ventricle. This is particularly evident when the exploring electrode is placed over the right ventricle. The hypertrophy of the right ventricle produces marked right axis deviation in the standard leads (page 101), the QRS complex is mainly positive in V_R and V_F and negative in V_L (Fig. 157). In the precordial leads recorded over the right ventricle the widened QRS complex is mainly positive in V_1 and the intrinsicoid deflection (page 195) is late, whereas in V_5 and V_6 recorded to the left of the transition zone, the R wave tends to be low, the intrinsicoid deflection early and the S wave wide, slurred and great

in amplitude (Fig. 157). Transitions in pattern from the normal configurations of the electrocardiogram (Fig. 169) to the typical pattern of
marked right ventricular hypertrophy (Fig. 157) develop with varying
degrees of right ventricular hypertrophy. The pattern shown in figure
157 is more likely to develop when the right ventricular hypertrophy is
due to pulmonary hypertension, *i.e.*, hypertrophy due to elevations in
pressure.

When increased work of the right ventricle is due to an increased
volume of output, hypertrophy of the crista supraventricularis develops
and the electrocardiographic pattern is fairly characteristic (Fig. 163).

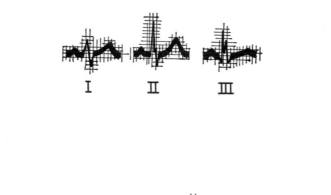

I   II   III

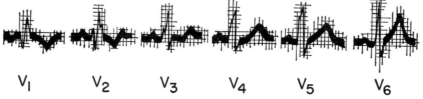

V_1 V_2 V_3 V_4 V_5 V_6

Fig. 163.—Characteristic changes in the QRS complex produced by congenital
interatrial septal defect of the secundum type. Such changes are usually produced
by a high volume output of the right ventricle and hypertrophy of the crista supraventricularis.

There is a prominent, wide and slurred S wave in lead I, a tendency to
right axis deviation of the QRS complex, a prominent, wide and slurred
terminal-positive deflection (R wave or R′ wave) in V_R, a wide, slurred
and prominent R or R′ wave in V_1 and a wide, slurred and prominent S
wave in V_5 and V_6 (Fig. 163). As the hypertrophy continues the QRS
complex widens further so that the pattern is often erroneously considered to represent incomplete or even complete right bundle branch
block. However, the gradual changes noted in several electrocardiograms
eliminate bundle branch block as the cause of the pattern. Such patterns
are common in congenital atrial septal defects of the secundum type.

In the primum type or with persistence of the atrioventricular canal the electrocardiographic pattern is the same except that the standard leads show left axis deviation (Fig. 164).

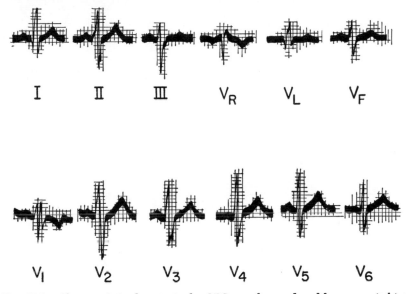

FIG. 164.—Characteristic changes in the QRS complex produced by congenital inter-atrial septal defect of the primum type. The changes are very similar to those shown in Fig. 163 except for the left axis deviation of the QRS complex.

Left Ventricular Hypertrophy

When the left ventricle is hypertrophied it has an even greater than normal influence over the right ventricle. The standard leads show the typical change of left ventricular hypertrophy (Page 136, Figs. 144 and 145). The QRS complex consists primarily of negative deflection of great amplitude in V_1 and a positive deflection of great amplitude in V_5 and V_6. J and the S–T segment are displaced below the isopotential line and the T wave is coved and inverted in V_5 and V_6 (Fig. 160). As the hypertrophy increases the QRS complex progressively widens and becomes more and more slurred and deformed so that the pattern is often erroneously considered to indicate incomplete or complete left bundle branch block (Fig. 165). Serially recorded electrocardiograms usually eliminate such errors.

MULTIPLE PRECORDIAL LEADS

When the precordial leads are recorded from different areas of the chest, *multiple precordial leads* are obtained. These series are sometimes

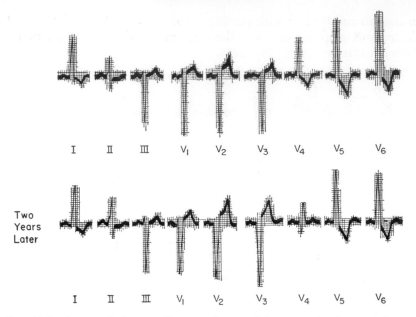

FIG. 165.—A typical electrocardiogram showing left ventricular hypertrophy with widening of the QRS complex to over 0.12 sec. within two years. Although the QRS complex exceeds 0.12 sec. in duration it does not represent left bundle branch block, but rather a thick ventricular wall which required a longer period of time to depolarize.

called the CF, CR, CL, CB or V leads. The *first letter* indicates that the exploring electrode is placed on the *chest;* the *second letter* indicates the location of the indifferent electrode. These sites are the same as those described previously for the single precordial leads. A numerical *subscript* following the second letter indicates the *exact* site on the chest where the exploring electrode is placed (Fig. 166). The sites are: (1) the fourth intercostal space at the right margin of the sternum; (2) the fourth intercostal space at the left margin of the sternum; (3) midway on the straight line connecting 2 and 4 electrode positions; (4) the fifth intercostal space at the left midclavicular line; (5) left anterior axillary line horizontally from position 4; (6) left midaxillary line at the same horizontal level as positions 4 and 5.

From what has been said, then, in a CF$_1$ lead the *exploring electrode* is placed on the chest in the fourth intercostal space at the right sternal margin (probably near the right ventricle or adjacent to the right atrium in the normal heart), and the *indifferent electrode* is placed on the left leg just above the ankle. A CR$_4$ lead indicates that the exploring electrode is in the fifth intercostal space in the left midclavicular line, which is usually just to the left of the apex of the normal heart, and the *indifferent electrode* is on the right arm. In both instances the connections are made so that when the exploring electrode is relatively positive with respect to the indifferent electrode, a positive deflection is inscribed on the electrocardiogram.

The connections are made as described early in this chapter for the single precordial leads. For example, when the CF_1 to CF_6 series of multiple leads is taken, the *LA electrode* is connected to the left leg just above the ankle, and the *LL electrode* is placed over the precordium in the successive positions as described for the subscripts above. The electrocardiograph is set at the lead III position as for recording the standard lead III.

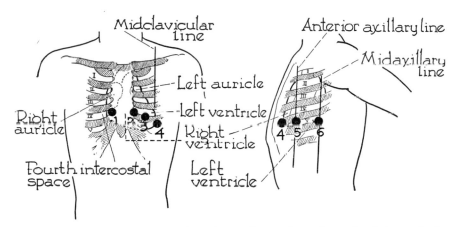

Fig. 166.—Points on the chest where the exploring electrode is placed for multiple precordial leads.

The electrocardiographs marketed today are wired to permit recording of the precordial and special leads by mere use of a selector switch and by placing the precordial electrode at the proper positions. The switch takes care of the connections and polarity of the electrodes. In avoidance of complex wiring and an elaborate switch, the self-contained switches are wired for recording the aV_R, aV_L, and AV_F leads but not V_R, V_L, and V_F. Because of certain advantages of the latter unipolar limb leads over the augmented ones, it is recommended that the switch be turned to the V position and the exploring precordial electrode be placed on the right and left arms and the left leg to record serially V_R, V_L, and V_F.

OTHER PRECORDIAL AND ESOPHAGEAL LEADS

It should be remembered that frequently, because of the position of the heart or the disease process, it is necessary to employ positions for the exploring electrode more to the right or left or above or below the usual six sites of the multiple chest leads. For example, it is necessary to place

11

the exploring electrode in the third interspace, or sixth interspace, or at the level of the ensiform cartilage, or in the left posterior axillary line, in order to localize sites of infarction or bundle branch block. The indications for such positions will become obvious after a study of this chapter.

If it is desired to determine the electric activity of the auricles or posterior wall of the ventricle, the exploring electrode is placed in the esophagus at the level at which the left auricle or ventricle rests against this organ (Fig. 167). In man this electrode is placed about as close to the heart of intact man as possible without surgical assistance. The *indifferent electrode* is placed as described previously.

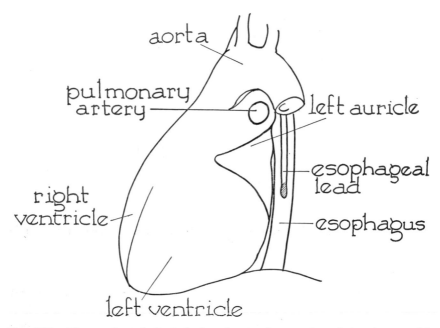

Fig. 167.—The esophageal electrode lies close to the auricle and therefore amplifies auricular electric activity.

The esophageal lead is used when it is impossible to identfy P waves in the standard leads, and it is especially desirable in the study of auricular depolarization. The P waves in the esophageal leads are usually peaked and of great amplitude (Fig. 168). This lead is also used to identify and study posterior myocardial infarction.

It is advisable first to attempt to record auricular activity by placing the exploring electrode in the third intercostal space at the right or left margin of the sternum before resorting to the use of the esophageal electrode positions. It is then near enough to the auricles to obtain definite P waves in most instances, if there is depolarization of the auricles. This is ordinarily sufficient to show the presence or absence of P waves. Considerable discomfort is encountered with passage into place of the esophageal electrode.

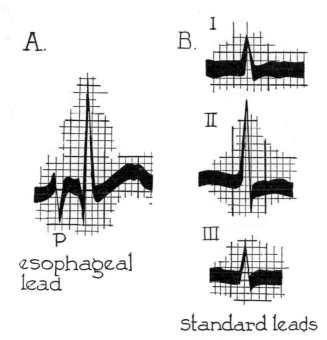

Fig. 168.—*A*, P waves as seen in the esophageal lead (the polarity of the esophageal electrode is reversed). *B*, No definite P wave could be identified in the standard leads.

THE CHARACTERISTICS OF THE NORMAL PRECORDIAL LEADS

Since the V leads are the most accurate, they should be employed generally, and discussions of multiple leads will be limited to them. Although some still consider the CF leads as satisfactory as the V leads, they are certainly not preferred. The arguments and characteristics presented below for the V leads hold more or less for the CF, CR or CL leads. In the latter, the indifferent electrode is not truly indifferent and therefore any quantitative analysis of these leads is difficult. Furthermore, it is not more difficult to record V leads than CF leads.

Although until recently, the most frequently employed single precordial lead in some was IVF. However, it is advantageous to record all six precordial leads (V_1 to V_6) when searching for small isolated lesions of the myocardium. Fortunately, the use of a single precordial lead has been discontinued almost entirely by those who understand electrocardiography. Normally, V_5 and V_6 resemble the standard lead I. The deflections in V_1 are often completely opposite to those in V_5 and V_6. It has a negative P wave and a negative or positive T wave, a small R and a large

S wave (Fig. 169). Lead V_4 is similar to lead 4V if the apex is in the fifth intercostal space near the midclavicular line. In the adult, the P wave is small, the R and S waves are about of equal size, and the T wave is positive in lead V_4 (Fig. 169). Transitional configurations between V_1 and V_6 are seen in leads V_2, V_3, V_4 and V_5. Leads V_5 and V_6 are like lead I. They show decreasing amplitude of the S waves (Fig. 169).

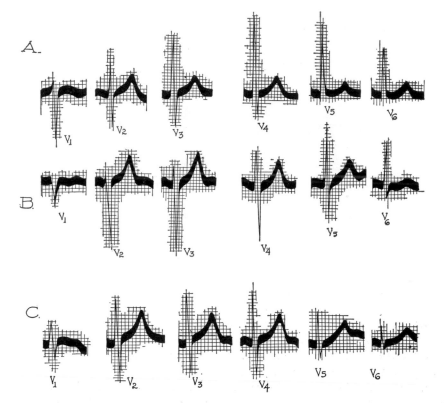

FIG. 169.—Normal variations in the six precordial leads. The "transition" zone is more to the right in group C, where R and S first become essentially equal in magnitude in V_2, and more to the left in group B, where R and S first become essentially equal in magnitude in V_4.

In V_1, V_2, and V_3, recorded with the exploring electrodes over the right ventricle, the R waves are relatively small and the S waves relatively large, since the depolarization process in the right ventricle, which is moving toward the exploring electrode, is associated with a relatively smaller electric potential than is the depolarization process moving away in the large mass of left ventricular musculature. Similarly, in the V_5 and V_6 leads, with the exploring electrodes over the left ventricle, the R waves are large and the S waves are small.

The transitional zone over the precordium refers to that electrocardiographic position in which the positive and negative (R and S) deflections of the QRS complex are essentially equal in amplitude, usually at the anterior interventricular groove. To the left of this transitional zone, *i.e.*, with the precordial electrode over the left ventricle, the main QRS deflection is positive, whereas to the right of this zone, or over the right ventricle, the main QRS deflection is negative (Fig. 169). Such localization of the transitional zone enables better evaluation of rotation about the longitudinal axis of the heart.

For more thorough exploration of the heart, the exploring electrode may be placed further to the left and around the chest at the same horizontal level as V_6, for example, V_7 in the left posterior axillary line, V_8 in the left midscapulary line, V_9 in the left paravertebral line, and so forth. The exploring electrode may also be placed in positions to the right of V_1, *i.e.*, V_4R position is located in the right midclavicular line at the same horizontal level as V_4, and V_3R is at the midpoint of a line connecting the positions of V_1 and V_4R. Leads V_3R and V_4R tend to resemble V_1. These leads to the right of V_1 and to the left of V_6 provide little assistance in clinical electrocardiography beyond that offered by the standard limb leads, unipolar limb leads, and precordial leads V_1 through V_6.

V_1 through V_6 may be recorded at the level of the third interspace, or at the level of the tip of the ensiform at the same longitudinal positions as V_1 through V_6 previously described, to explore the basal and lateral and the apical and lower anterior and inferior aspects of the heart, respectively.

The description of the components of the electrocardiogram immediately below will be confined to lead 4V, unless otherwise stated, for whenever a single precordial V lead is recorded, it is the one most commonly employed today. The nomenclature of the components of the completed tracings of all chest or special leads is the same as described in the previous chapter for the standard leads. The differences are noted for the chest leads in this and other chapters to follow.

The characteristics of the various portions of lead 4V are as follows:

The P Wave

The P wave is normally diphasic $(- +)$ or inverted and, less commonly, upright in the adult.

The P–R Interval

This is not significantly different from that described for the standard leads.

The QRS Complex

The QRS complex is slightly wider than in the standard leads, reaching 0.12 second normally in some people.

The Q Wave

A small Q wave is present in a small percentage of 4V leads. The duration is from 0.01 to 0.02 second, and the amplitude is usually not greater than 0.2 millimeter. A Q_1 wave is usually associated with a Q wave in lead 4V.

The R Wave

The amplitude of the normal R wave usually varies from 2 to 22 millimeters (averages about 11 millimeters). If the R wave is less than 1 millimeter, anterior myocardial infarction immediately under the exploring electrode is highly probable.

The S Wave

The S wave varies from 0 to 20 millimeters (averages about 10 millimeters) in amplitude. If the electrode is far to the left, the S wave is often absent.

The S–T Segment

The segment is short or absent, since repolarization normally begins before depolarization is complete; the exploring electrode is near the heart so that the small amounts of current associated with early repolarization are recorded when they are often not recorded in the standard leads. This results in shifting of the segment and of J, the normal shift varying between −1 to +3 millimeters. The segment is shifted upward in anterior infarction. With left ventricular hypertrophy the segment is shifted downward when the electrode is over the left ventricle and upward when it is over the right ventricle.

Digitalis and the related group of drugs often produce a shift of J and the S–T segment. The shift is opposite to the main initial deflection of the QRS, with a tendency for the S–T segment to be straight and not rounded. The effects are similar to those described in Chapter 2 for lead I.

The T Wave

The amplitude of the T wave ranges from 1 to 13 millimeters, averaging 5 millimeters in females and 7 millimeters in males. The T wave is always upright in the adult if the electrode is properly placed, *i.e.*, over or slightly to the left of the apex. In the child the wave is often inverted (60 per cent of children in some series). If the electrode is placed to the left and upward in the fourth intercostal space, an upright wave is often obtained in the child. Precordial leads in children should probably be recorded in this position routinely. The negative wave in 4V in the child is probably attributable to the fact that near the apex the direction of the repolarization process occurs from the endocardial surface to the epicardial surface instead of in reverse order, as in the adult. The age at which the T wave in the child becomes upright is unknown. Subjects of twenty-one years of age or more, rarely, if ever, have a negative T wave in lead 4V, if it is at or to the left of the transitional zone, and, in fact, such a negative wave is indicative of myocardial disease, provided the precordial electrode is properly placed. *The normal T wave in the adult* is rarely notched or diphasic. The T wave is inverted in patients with anterior infarction and in patients with anterolateral ischemia of the heart. The T wave in 4V is often inverted when T_1 is inverted.

The U Wave

The U wave is often inverted in disease states, frequently rendering measurement of the Q–T interval difficult. Its significance is the same as that described for the standard leads.

Slurring and Notching

Mild degrees of notching are frequently present normally. Extreme slurring of the upstroke of the R wave is often abnormal and will be considered under bundle branch block. Slight slurring of the waves of the QRS group occurs normally.

CLINICAL APPLICATIONS OF THE CHEST LEADS

Complete Right Bundle Branch Block

Supraventricular impulses flowing through the bundle of His pass into the bundle branches. Impulses passing down the right bundle branch are blocked in complete right bundle branch block, whereas those passing down the left branch activate the left ventricle in the usual manner. In right BBB the impulses traveling down the intact left bundle traverse the septum, which requires at least 0.04 second, and are distributed to the right ventricle by means of the Purkinje system. The entire time for the recording of the QRS complex is always greater than 0.12 second for cardiac rates of 70 or less. The time required to activate the right ventricle is increased and the path over which the depolarization process traversed is aberrant (see Chapter 2, BBB in the standard leads). Thus, if an electrode were placed over the right ventricle, *i.e.*, for leads V_1 and V_2, that portion of the QRS complex with the greatest duration would be upright and slurred (Fig. 170).

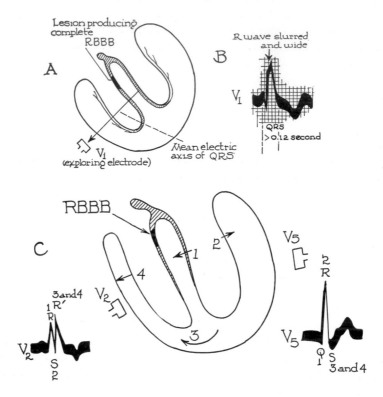

Fɪɢ. 170.—*A*, Since the depolarization process is traveling *slowly* toward the precordial electrode of lead V_1, a wide upward deflection is inscribed, the electrode being positive during the greater part of depolarization. *B*, Because of the duration and aberrant route, the wave is also wide, slurred and variously deformed. Part *C* shows the mechanism by which the "bifid" R develops in a unipolar lead recorded with the precordial electrode over the right ventricle. The impulse first depolarizes the septum from the left (force 1), producing a small R wave. Next, the thick wall of the left ventricle begins to be depolarized (force 2), producing an S wave. These two processes are essentially normal in their order. Then the impulse migrates around the apex in an abnormal fashion (force 3), approaching the right side of the heart and the precordial electrode. This produces a slurred R wave. Finally, the free wall of the right ventricle is depolarized (force 4), terminating the event. The resultant "bifid" R is shown in lead V_2.

When the electrode is placed over the left ventricle, *i.e.*, for lead V_5 or V_6, the major deflection (one of greatest duration) of the QRS complex is negative and deformed as the aberrant depolarization process progresses away from the V_5 or V_6 precordial electrode (Fig. 171).

At times, it is necessary to record precordial leads with the exploring electrode farther to the right and left than for the V_1 and V_6 leads, in order to bring out the foregoing characteristics. In RBBB a bifid R wave (in V_1 and V_2 of Fig. 170 and in V_2 and V_3 of Fig. 172) is usually seen in one of the leads recorded from a region over the right ventricle, whereas in LBBB a bifid R wave (R, R') is encountered in one of the precordial leads recorded over the left ventricle.

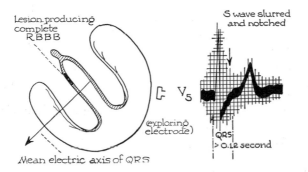

Fig. 171.—The precordial electrode of lead V_5 or V_6 over the left ventricle and the resultant tracing. The deflection of greatest duration is down, as the exploring electrode is relatively negative during the greater part of ventricular depolarization. Since the pathway is abnormal, its deflection is slurred and deformed.

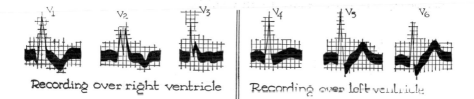

Fig. 172.—The chest leads in *right BBB*. The exploring electrode is placed over the right ventricle (V_1 and V_2) and over the left ventricle (V_5 and V_6).

Complete Left Bundle Branch Block

In complete *left BBB* the mechanisms producing the electrogradiographic patterns are essentially the reverse of those for RBBB. The impulse is blocked in the left bundle branch and the depolarization process is delayed and aberrant, since it passes through the septum from the right ventricle to the left ventricle. As a result, the major deflection, *i.e.*, the one of greatest duration of the QRS complex, is downward or negative when the exploring electrode is placed over the right ventricle (V_1 and V_2) and upward or positive when the exploring electrode is placed over the left ventricle (V_5 and V_6, Fig. 173). The duration of the entire QRS complex is again always greater than 0.12 second.

The P waves and P–R intervals indicate that one is dealing with complete BBB and not an ectopic mechanism. Needless to say, it is necessary to determine accurately the pathway of the impulse in identifying BBB (see Chapter 2).

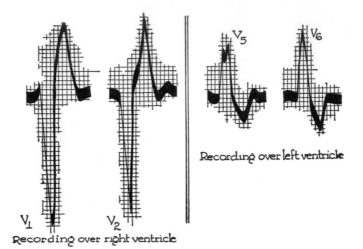

Fig. 173.—*Left BBB,* showing the wide (main) *negative* deflections with the exploring electrode over the right ventricle and the wide (main) *positive* deflections with the exploring electrode over the left ventricle.

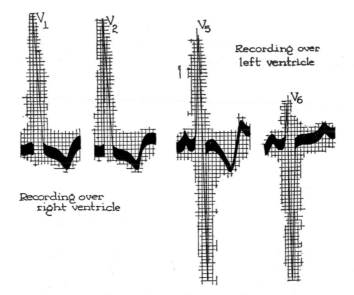

Fig. 174.—The chest leads in right axis deviation. (See text for explanation.)

Axis Deviation

The picture of *right axis deviation* is essentially that of right BBB. The major deflection of the QRS complex is the one of greatest amplitude; as for the standard leads, it would be a great deal more correct if areas under the deflections rather than amplitude were used for these measurements. It is positive or upright when the exploring electrode is placed over the right ventricle and negative or down when the exploring electrode is placed over the left ventricle (Fig. 174). The width of these QRS complexes is essentially normal.

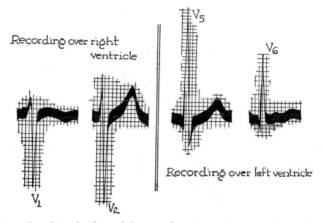

FIG. 175.—The chest leads in left axis deviation. (See text for explanation.)

The pattern of *left axis deviation* is essentially the reverse of that seen in right axis deviation. The deflection of greatest amplitude of the QRS complex is down or negative when the exploring electrode is placed over the right ventricle (V_1 and V_2) and upward or positive when the exploring electrode is placed over the left ventricle (V_5 and V_6) (Fig. 175). The S wave in V_1 and V_2 and the R wave in V_5 and V_6 are usually of larger magnitude than in the normal chest leads.

Myocardial Infarction

Myocardial infarcts have been divided into those which occur at the *endocardial surface* of the heart, those at the *epicardial surface* of the heart, and those *within the myocardium* itself (*intramural*). *Transmural* infarcts are essentially a combination of the first two. It has been pointed out that intramural infarcts (Fig. 139) exert electric effects equally in all directions and hence do not create a potential difference measurable by the electrocardiograph. Infarcts located at the epicardial or endocardial surfaces, however, do create measurable electric changes.

It has also been stated that the muscle adjacent to the *infarcted area is polarized in a manner to appear as though the negative charges* are within the injured area and the *positive charges are outside the injured zone* but within the zone of ischemia (Chapter 2). It is the relationship between the potential differences produced by the infarcted area, those produced by the remaining normal portion of the heart, and the relative position of the precordial electrode that determines the configuration of the completed electrocardiogram in the chest leads. The forces concerned with the three zones related to the infarct have been discussed in detail

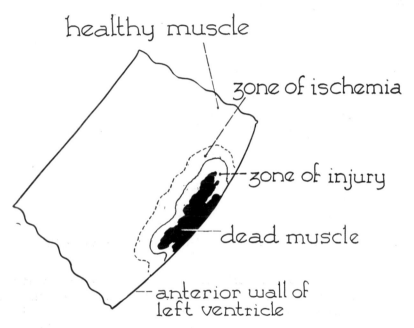

Fig. 176.—A section through the anterior wall of the left ventricle, showing the important physiologic zones of an infarct situated at the epicardial surface of the heart. Remember that these zones are really "shells," since they occur in three-dimensional space.

in Chapter 2 and will not be repeated here. It is important to review this discussion carefully before attempting a study of the presentation to follow, which concerns the use of the precordial leads in the diagnosis and localization of myocardial infarction.

Anterior Myocardial Infarction.—One of the most important rôles played by the chest leads is in the diagnosis and management of myocardial infarction, particularly of the left or anterolateral wall of the heart. They usually appear at the anterolateral surface of the left ventricle and the adjacent part of the septum (Fig. 125). When occlusion of a portion of the left coronary artery occurs, that part of the myocardium irrigated

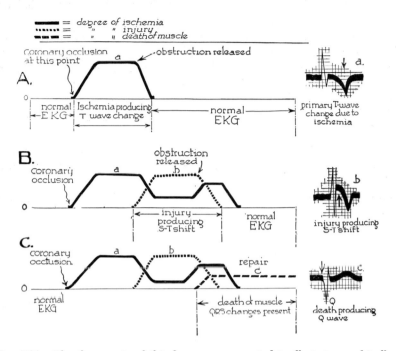

Fig. 177.—The three parts of this figure are presented to illustrate graphically the temporal relationships of the electrocardiographic changes encountered in any precordial lead recorded with the exploring electrode placed over and near an area of myocardial infarction. Anterolateral myocardial infarction is discussed in particular, since it is so common and since the exploring electrode can be placed so readily over, and certainly near, the area of infarction. The same argument can be applied to the changes in any type of properly recorded chest lead. In fact, with some reservations, they are applicable to the standard leads as well.

Part A shows the effects of temporary obstruction of a coronary artery with temporary ischemia of the myocardium subjacent to the exploring electrode; *a* represents T wave change during the ischemic period.

Parts B and C.—The course of the changes in the electrocardiogram in infarction subjacent to the exploring electrode. Part B.—If the occlusion lasts a longer period of time, the ischemia results in injury to the myocardium, thus producing *not only* ischemic changes (T wave changes) but changes due to currents of injury (shifts in the S–T segment) indicated by an elevation of the S–T segment. If the occlusion is released before permanent damage results, the electrocardiogram returns to normal.

Part C.—If the occlusion persists a long period of time, *not only* are ischemic changes (T wave inversion) and current of injury effects (elevation of the S–T segment) recorded, but in addition effects due to dead muscle, QRS changes (usually a low R wave, less than 1 millimeter, or an absence of an R wave) result. Once death of muscle occurs, release of the occlusion is only of partial benefit. As repair takes place, the current of injury effects (S–T segment elevation) disappear first, the ischemic effects (T wave inversion) may disappear much later, and the death of muscle changes (absence of R wave) are last, if ever, to vanish.

The type of tracing that would be recorded from a position over the infarct at the various periods is indicated and labeled *a*, *b*, and *c*. Each would be recorded at the time indicated by *a*, *b*, and *c* on the graph. These changes, in man, take place in a matter of seconds, minutes, hours or days.

by it undergoes certain changes which are illustrated in figure 176. These may be summarized as follows:

Occlusion first produces an area of *ischemia* which is of short duration and is soon *replaced by injured muscle,* capable of producing currents of injury. If the occlusion persists, the central portion of the injured area dies and a series of "shells" of muscle remain, as indicated by figure 176.

The *zone of dead muscle (dead zone)* is mainly responsible for the low, or absent, R wave or Q wave when the precordial or exploring electrode is placed over the infarcted area.

The *zone of injured muscle (injured zone)* is responsible for shifts in the S–T segment (see Chapters 1 and 2 and the discussion of infarction in the standard leads).

The *zone of ischemia (ischemic zone)* is responsible for changes in the T waves (Chapter 2).

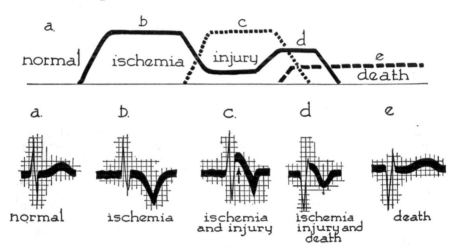

Fig. 178.—Changes in the electrocardiographic pattern in which a precordial lead was placed directly over an area of myocardial infarction. Tracing *b* is seen early after infarction and *e* many weeks afterwards.

The progressive changes which take place following occlusion may be illustrated by figure 177 (modified from R. H. Bayley).

If the electrocardiograms are collected during the first few seconds or even hours after occlusion and if the exploring electrode is placed over the area of infarction, the picture of acute anterior infarction may be seen (Fig. 178*b*). At first there is ischemia, so that only inversion of the T wave is present. This may be fleeting and is often not detected clinically. A few hours later the ischemic area is altered and is sufficiently injured to produce currents of injury. As the area of injury increases in size, the area of ischemia decreases. At this point there is elevation of the S–T segment with or without extreme inversion of the T wave (Fig. 178*c*). If the occlu-

sion persists until death of muscle within the injured area ensues, a Q
wave appears and the R wave decreases in amplitude or completely disappears (Fig. 178*d*). After a period of days or weeks, the injured area
recovers, usually preceding disappearance of the ischemic area. At this
time the S–T segment returns to the isoelectric line, leaving no R wave,
but a Q (QS) wave and inverted T wave to indicate the presence of the
infarct (Fig. 178*d*). The latter picture represents the chronic stage, which
may last many months. As the ischemic area gradually recovers, the T
wave becomes upright and often the only sign of a previous infarct is the
absence of an R wave (Fig. 178*e*).

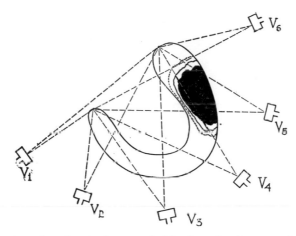

Fig. 179.—The value of multiple precordial leads in the diagnosis of localized areas
of muscle death is shown. Leads V_1, V_2 and V_3 are influenced relatively slightly, as
they are far from and lateral to the infarct. Leads V_4, V_5 and V_6 each are influenced
to a greater extent by the infarct. The potential represented by the angle subtended
by the infarct is negative in V_5. This results in a low amplitude or absence of the R
wave in this lead. The solid angles from the margins of the infarct are not depicted in
this figure.

The advantages of multiple precordial leads over a single one is generally recognized. If the precordial leads are placed in relation to the infarcted heart as shown in figure 179, and the infarct is in the anterolateral
region of the left ventricle, it can be seen that the infarcted area will vary
in its influence upon the exploring electrode, depending upon its position.
The effect of the infarct on any one precordial lead will also depend upon
the proximity of the exploring electrode to the infarct and upon the size of
the infarct (Fig. 179). Since the depolarization of the wall of the heart
subjacent to the exploring electrode produces the R wave, it follows that
the R wave will be completely absent or greatly reduced in amplitude
when the apex is sufficiently infarcted, if the exploring electrode is over
the infarcted area (see V_5, Fig. 179). The mechanism for these changes
can be explain by figure 179.

It is possible to predict with a great deal of accuracy the effects of the infarcts on the QRS complex of any given chest lead. The magnitude of the potential at the exploring electrode in use may be represented by an angle located at the electrode, with its sides subtended by the margins of the atrioventricular orifices (Fig. 180). This potential in the case of the exploring electrode of V_5 is the algebraic sum of strong positive forces from the nearby wall of the thick left ventricle and the weaker negative forces exerted by the more distant wall of the thinner right ventricle. The major effect of these two forces is a positive initial deflection in the QRS

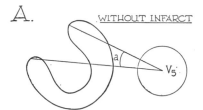

A.   WITHOUT INFARCT

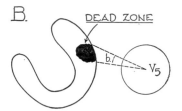

B.   DEAD ZONE

Solid angle (a) subtended at V_5 by atrio-ventricular orifices of ventricles. The force is positive and arbitrarily considered +4units

Solid angle (b) subtended by epicardial margins of the infarct. Effect is to reduce the positive force exerted by left ventricle. This is arbitrarily taken to indicate a loss of 3 positive units of potential

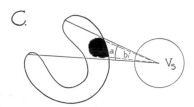

C.

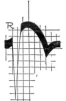

Algebraic effect of solid angles (a) and (b) is a force of +1.

Small upright R wave of 1 unit will be written in Lead V_5

Resultant effect of forces represented by angles (a) and (b) is a positive force of 1 unit exerted at V_5

Fig. 180.—The amplitude and direction of the R wave may be predicted from the algebraic sum of the solid angles from the atrioventricular orifices of the ventricles and the infarcted area. (See text for details.)

complex of V_5 in the normal heart (Fig. 180A). If there is a moderately large infarct with resulting death of a moderately large mass of muscle in the left ventricle immediately subjacent to the exploring electrode, this results in a loss of most, if not all, of the positive force offered normally by the left ventricle (Fig. 180B). The negative force exerted by the still normal opposite wall almost predominates and, therefore, there is only a small, positive deflection initially in the completed electrocardiogram of V_5 a small R wave (Fig. 180B).

The effect of a larger infarct is to produce a large *"physiologic hole"* in the heart. For example, in figure 181 the large infarct completely elimi-nates the positive force exerted by the left ventricle at the infarcted area, and the negative force from the opposite wall is unneutralized. Its effect on the electrocardiogram in V_5 is to produce a large initial downward deflection, a *QS wave*, with absence of an R wave (Fig. 181).

It is obvious from what has been said that *in patients with myocardial infarction, when the exploring electrode is placed over the infarcted area, the R wave is usually absent*, and its absence is indicative of death of muscle.

An R wave may be recorded in the presence of infarction if the infarct is intramural, if it is small, or if it is in certain regions, such as high at the base of the heart, where it influences the exploring electrode little.

As in the standard leads, the direction of the electric force responsible for the S–T shift is indicated by a "vector" drawn from the centroid of the ventricles to the centroid of the infarcted area, the head of the arrow being relatively positive. If this electric force is directed toward the precordial electrode, that is, if the precordial electrode is relatively positive, the S–T segment is shifted upward and if away from the exploring electrode, the shift is negative or downward (Fig. 182). In subendocardial infarcts the forces act in an opposite direction, for obvious reasons.

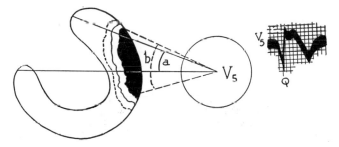

Fig. 181.—The R wave is absent when the angle subtended by the infarct is larger than that subtended by the atrioventricular orifices of the ventricles. A downward deflection (Q) is written.

If the exploring electrode is placed directly over the infarct, the apex of the T wave will be opposite in direction to the shift of the S–T segment, as electric forces developed during repolarization of the ventricle are directed opposite to those responsible for the shift of the S–T segment. For example, in an anterior infarct involving the apex of the heart, we find the three zones produced by the infarct as indicated in figure 183. In the zone of ischemia the repolarization process is delayed so that repolarization begins, in the area of the heart immediately below the exploring electrode at the area of infarction, from the endocardial surface instead of from the epicardial surface as it does normally. This effects a field of relative negativity at the exploring electrode. The vector force produced by this field is indicated by a', figure 183. The solid angle subtended by the repolarization process is essentially as indicated by the

12

sides *a*, figure 183. The repolarization process in the remaining portion of the heart also creates a negative field about the exploring electrode. This force is represented by the solid angle subtended at the exploring electrode by the margins of the atrioventricular orifices. The sides of this angle are labeled *b*, and the vector force is represented by *b'*, figure 183. These two negative forces create a relatively strong negative field about the exploring electrode during the process of repolarization.

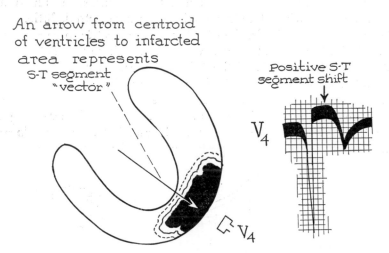

An arrow from centroid of ventricles to infarcted area represents S-T segment "vector"

Positive S·T segment shift

V_4

V_4

Fig. 182.—*The S–T segment shift* is positive when a "vector" drawn from the centroid of the ventricles to the centroid of the infarcted area points toward the precordial electrode. The S–T segment is shifted upward in anterior myocardial infarction when the precordial electrode is placed immediately over the infarcted area.

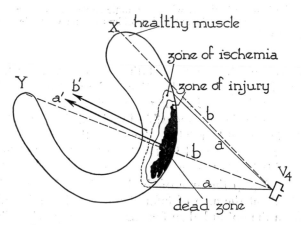

X healthy muscle

zone of ischemia

zone of injury

Y   *b'*   *a'*

b

b

a

V_4

dead zone

Fig. 183.—*X* and *Y* represent portions of the left and right ventricles. The infarcted area in the epicardial region near the apex of the left ventricle with its various shells or zones is indicated. The mechanisms responsible for the forces acting on the exploring electrode are discussed in the text. The vector forces *a'* and *b'* are responsible for the inscription of the T wave in the completed electrocardiogram in lead V_4.

Posterior Myocardial Infarction.—The precordial leads are of less practical value in the diagnosis of posterior infarction than anterior infarction. In some cases the S–T segment is depressed, and the T wave is tall. Since the infarct is usually in the diaphragmatic, posterior, and septal portion of the left and right ventricles, and the apex is not involved, the R wave is not abnormal. A vector force drawn from the centroid of the ventricle to the infarcted area is directed away from the precordial electrode; hence the S–T shift is downward. The vector representing the electric force responsible for the T wave is directed opposite to the vector representing the electric force responsible for the S–T segment shift (Figs. 183 and 184).

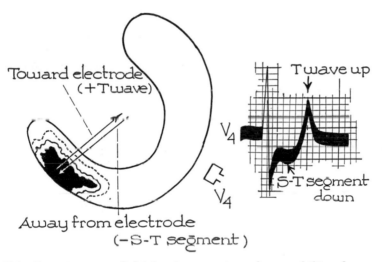

Fig. 184.—Posterior myocardial infarction sometimes shows a shifting downward of the S–T segment. The T wave is upright and is of increased amplitude.

It should be pointed out that various combinations may be obtained when more than one infarct has occurred or when infarction and some other disease state, such as pericarditis, exist simultaneously. The effects of the most recent and of the largest injury tend to predominate in the completed electrocardiogram. The closer the infarct is to the exploring electrode, the greater is its effect on the electrocardiogram.

LOCALIZING INFARCTS RATHER PRECISELY

From the preceding discussion about anterior and posterior infarction, it is seen that the position of the exploring electrode in relation to the infarcted area will determine the electrocardiographic pattern in that precordial lead. By means of extensive and adequate exploration of the cardiac region of the chest to record many leads and by a study of the resultant tracing in each lead, the infarcted area can be localized fairly sharply. Several examples will be discussed here.

Anteroseptal Infarction

In infarction of the anteroseptal region the changes in the precordial leads tend to be confined to tracings taken over the right side of the heart, namely, V_2 and V_3, and to some extent V_1 and V_4, as the exploring elec-

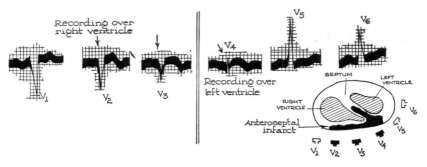

FIG. 185.—Anteroseptal infarction.

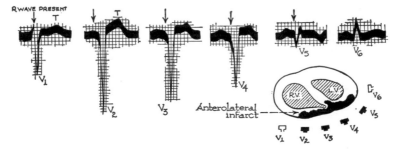

FIG. 186.—*Anterolateral infarction.* The R wave is absent, the S–T segment elevated, and the T wave negative in the precordial leads in which the exploring electrode is placed in the 2nd, 3rd, 4th and 5th precordial positions. In the 1st and 6th positions, an R wave is present. Such an infarct must be in the *anterolateral* position.

trodes in these leads are over or near the infarcted area. In these leads the pattern is the same as described previously for anterior infarction with the exploring electrode placed over the area of infarction. The changes in V_5 and V_6 are not characteristic and may be limited to the T wave (Fig. 185). The reasons for such findings can be found in the previous discussions.

Anterolateral Infarction

In anterolateral infarction (Fig. 186) the diagnostic signs of infarction will be displayed by leads V_3, V_4, and V_5 and perhaps also by V_1, V_2, and

V_6 if the infarct is extensive. In V_6 the R wave is more likely to be small than absent, and the T wave is likely to be of low amplitude and negative. Lead I usually shows the Q_1T_1 pattern, and V_L usually presents the QT pattern of infarction.

High Lateral (Basal) Infarction

In high lateral infarction it is possible that the usual precordial leads will show no diagnostic change of infarction, for the exploring electrode is likely not to be near enough to the infarcted area. The standard leads and V_L are likely to indicate the existence of infarction. However, if the precordial leads are moved up one or two intercostal spaces, the characteristic pattern will be recorded.

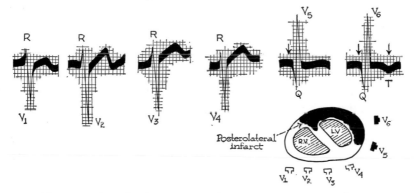

FIG. 187.—Posterolateral infarction. High T waves are present only in V_2, V_3 and V_4 because of the infarct in the posterior wall opposite to the exploring electrodes but not opposite to the exploring electrodes of leads V_5 and V_6. V_5 and V_6 show the typical pattern produced by an infarct in the wall immediately subjacent to the exploring electrodes of these leads.

Posterolateral Infarction

In *posterolateral infarction* (Fig. 187) the standard leads and V_F suggest posterior infarction, whereas the typical changes in the precordial leads are seen only in V_5 and V_6. In these latter two leads the QS wave is apt to be prominent, and the T waves are likely to be sharply inverted. In V_1 to V_4 the R and T waves are often unusually prominent.

Postero-inferior Infarction

In *postero-inferior infarction* (Fig. 188) the standard leads and V_F usually present the pattern of a posterior infarct, whereas the usual precordial leads will show nothing of significance. Diagnostic changes may be detected in EV_2. In this lead the exploring electrode is placed at the level of the tip of the ensiform cartilage in the left sternal line. The exploring electrode in EV₂ is more or less over the postero-inferior surface of the heart, where electric effects from the inferior surface of the heart may be recorded. The R wave is absent, the S–T segment tends to be shifted upward, and the T wave is sharply inverted in lead EV₂. In V₁ and V₂ the R wave is sometimes small if the area of infarction extends over the apical region of the heart.

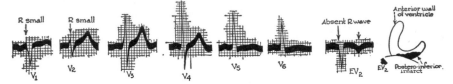

Fig. 188.—Postero-inferior infarction. Note the characteristic changes in lead EV₂ indicated by the arrows. Diagram to the right is a vertical section of the heart with the infarct.

Strictly Anterior Infarction

In *strictly anterior infarction* (Fig. 189) the standard leads or unipolar limb leads present no diagnostic pattern in infarction and may be entirely normal. In the multiple precordial leads the pattern of an anterior infarct is limited to V₂, V₃ and probably V₁ and/or V₄. V₁ is likely to show a low R wave and slight T wave changes. V₅ and V₆ are usually normal. The electrocardiographic pattern is essentially the same as for the anteroseptal infarct.

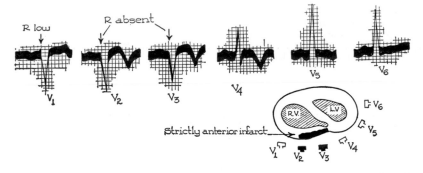

Fig. 189.—Strictly anterior infarction. The changes of infarction are found in those precordial leads in which the exploring electrode is immediately over the infarct, such as in V₂ and V₃.

Strictly Posterior Infarction

This has been discussed earlier in this presentation as posterior infarction.

It can be seen from the previous discussion that it is possible to localize an infarct fairly precisely with the use of the usual multiple pre-

cordial leads. If the infarct is diffuse, changes diagnostic of infarction
will be present in most, if not all, of the multiple precordial leads. If
more areas of the chest are explored, even on the posterior surface and
upper portions (third interspace), it is possible to localize most of the
infarcts in a patient with a typical clinical picture of infarction.

*There is a greater need to consider the term exploring electrode literally
and actually to explore the various regions of the heart in order to locate
precisely the site of infarction and to estimate its size. When infarction
is suspected, search should be made from area to area until the surface of
the heart has been explored thoroughly.*

HIGH BASAL INFARCTION

As indicated on pages 116 and 243 and in Figure 193, areas of the heart
which are depolarized last, such as the high basal portion of the left
ventricle, would not be expected to produce alterations in the early
portions of the QRS complex, *i.e.* they would not be expected to produce
Q wave changes, but rather to alter the late portions of the QRS complex.
These changes are reflected by notches and slurs of the late portions in
most, but not necessarily in all, leads. The deformities are usually most
evident in V_4, V_5 and/or V_6 and recognized best in serially recorded
tracings. The same types of abnormalities are produced in the midtemporal portions of the QRS complex when areas of the myocardium which
are depolarized in the midtemporal periods of ventricular depolarization
are infarcted.

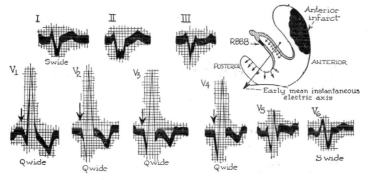

Fig. 190.—The changes in V_1 to V_6 produced by anteroseptal infarction complicated
by complete right BBB. The arrows indicate the large and wide Q waves in V_1, V_2, V_3
and V_4. The branch block does not interfere with the manifestations of the initial QRS
changes. Consult the text for reasons.

Infarction Complicated by Right Bundle Branch Block

The diagnostic pattern of infarction (located mainly in the left ventricle) in the limb leads is not greatly modified by the presence of right
BBB. This is also essentially true for the precordial leads. Because
depolarization and repolarization of the left ventricle occur in a normal

fashion in RBBB, the early portion of the QRS is inscribed in a more or less normal fashion, and therefore the electrocardiogram presents evidence of both RBBB and infarction (Fig. 190).

If there is *posterior infarction* in the *presence of RBBB*, the electrocardiographic pattern will present the signs of both, *i.e.*, the RBBB signs will not obscure the picture of infarction in the chest leads or in the limb leads.

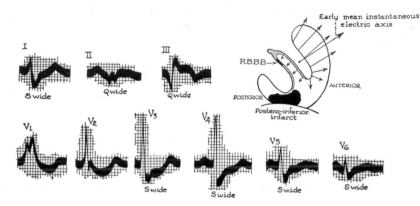

Fig. 191.—The changes in the standard limb leads and precordial leads in posterior-inferior infarction complicated by complete right BBB. The development of the typical deep and broad Q₃ wave is not disturbed by the branch block. Consult the text for reasons.

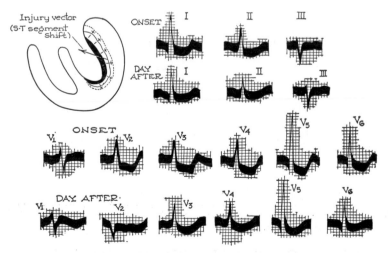

Fig. 192.—The changes in the standard limb leads and precordial leads in *subendo-cardial infarction* of the anterolateral wall of the left ventricle. The vector produced by the zone of injury and responsible for the S–T segment shift is directed from the centroid of the zone of infarction to the centroid of the heart, *i.e.*, "against the rule." This results in a depression of S–T in lead I and in the precordial leads recorded with the precordial electrode over the infarcted zone.

Infarction Complicated by Left Bundle Branch Block

This cardiac state is not likely to show anything except the picture of the LBBB, because the initial and the entire QRS complex are disturbed by the block, making it impossible for the pattern of infarction to manifest itself.

Subendocardial Infarction

Subendocardial infarction results in a reversal of the polarity of the vector force produced by the current of injury, that is, a shift "against the rule" of the S–T segments results in the completed electrocardiogram. The mechanism is illustrated in Figure 192.

PAPILLARY MUSCLE INFARCTION

In most instances, when the electrocardiogram shows the changes of subendocardial infarction the papillary muscles of the left ventricle are infarcted. Because of the anatomic orientation of the papillary muscle, large posteroseptal infarcts usually involve the posteromedial papillary muscle, whereas large anteroseptal infarcts usually include the antero-lateral papillary muscle. When the papillary muscle alone is infarcted or scarred, the electrocardiogram shows the signs of subendocardial infarction. Infarction of the posteromedial papillary muscle usually produces changes in leads recorded to the right of the transition zone (V_1 through V_4), whereas infarction of the anterolateral papillary muscle produces the changes in the leads recorded to the left of the transition zone (V_4 through V_6).

Temporal Relationships of the Depolarization Process to the Electrocardiogram

Lesions may be located anywhere in the heart. Those in areas normally depolarized early in the electric cycle would alter the early phases of the depolarization process whereas lesions in areas normally depolarized later in the electric cycle would alter later phases of the depolarization process. Therefore, infarctions discussed previously produce Q and QS waves or changes in the early portions of the QRS complex because the infarcts are localized to portions of the myocardium which are depolarized early (Figs. 126, 136, 186, 187). However, lesions localized to areas of the myocardium which are depolarized later in the electric cycle would not be expected to reflect alterations in the early portions of the QRS complex to produce characteristic Q or QS waves. Instead, notching, slurring and other distortions develop in later portions of the QRS complex (Fig. 193). For example, Figure 193a shows a process of depolarization which has spread for only 0.04 seconds. The wave front encountered an area of infarction early in the depolarization process which resulted in alterations in early portions of the QRS com-

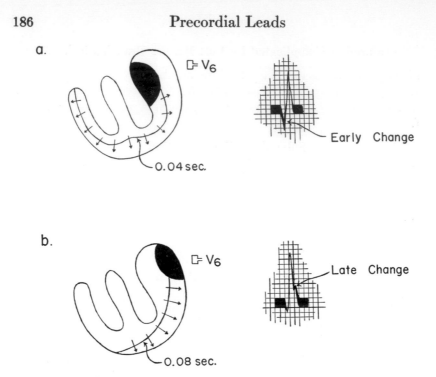

F𝗂𝗀. 193.—Infarcts in the myocardium encountered early, *a*, and later, *b*, by the depolarization process. When encountered early, *a*, the first phases of the QRS complex were altered resulting in a wide and deep Q wave. When encountered later, *b*, the downstroke of the QRS complex was deformed or notched but no Q or QS wave was produced.

plex, producing a wide Q wave in this instance. Figure 193*b* shows the wave front of the depolarization process later in the electric cycle in which an area of infarction was not encountered until 0.08 seconds after the depolarized process was under way. The lesion altered the time course of depolarization later in the electric cycle resulting in a notch on the downstroke of the QRS complex rather than a Q or QS wave.

Alterations in the QRS complex cannot be expected to occur until the lesion has had an opportunity to change the time course of the depolarization process. Therefore, it is necessary to consider the temporal relationship of the time course of the electrophysiologic phenomenon in the heart with its reflections in the electrocardiogram.

ANGINA PECTORIS

Angina pectoris may produce any of the changes listed for coronary occlusion (Chapter 2) except the QRS changes of infarction. It is obvious that the degree and duration of occlusion will determine whether the individual will have myocardial infarction or myocardial ischemia. The changes produced in patients with angina pectoris are usually seen during the bout of pain and ischemia and may be precipitated by exercise. These changes quickly disappear, to be seen again when the pain and ischemia return. It is possible for the electrocardiogram of a patient to manifest only T wave changes, or T wave changes and segment shifts, as occur with infarction. In angina pectoris the transient changes in the T waves and S–T segments occur in the standard leads as well. The diagnosis of *angina pectoris* is favored by the fact that these signs of ischemia or injury are noted, being present only for the duration of the pain, and by the rapid reversion of the electrocardiogram to the pattern present prior to the onset of the attack. The diagnostic electrocardiographic patterns are not so evanescent in infarction; they persist for hours, days, months, or even years. QRS changes are not characteristically present in angina pectoris as they are in coronary occlusion (Chapter 2).

PERICARDITIS

In figure 140 it was pointed out that the electric effects of pericarditis are usually due to a diffuse area of myocardial inflammation surrounding the ventricles of the heart subjacent to the pericarditis. A line drawn from the centroid of the ventricles to the centroid of the injured area, when transposed as a vector to the triaxial reference system, may be used to indicate the direction of the S–T *segment shifts* in the standard leads. When this vector is directed toward the overlying precordial electrodes,

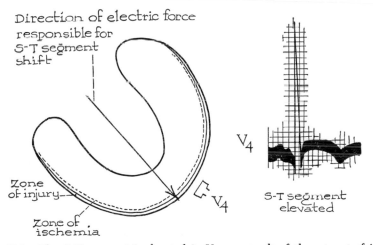

FIG. 194.—The S–T segment is elevated in V₄ as a result of the current of injury produced by the diffuse area of muscle injury subjacent to the pericarditis. The *actual* current of injury runs from the apex to the base of the heart but the *apparent* effect is as shown from the base to the apex. The apparent or visible effect is due to the current introduced by means of the battery in the control box. It is simple to visualize only small or no shifts in the S–T segments in V₁ and V₆. The direction of the electric force responsible for the S–T segment shifts is determined by drawing a "vector" from the centroid of the heart to the centroid of the injured zone with the positive end of the "vector" in the injured zone.

an upward displacement of the S–T segment in these leads will take place (Fig. 194). The arguments presented for the S–T segment and T wave changes apply for pericarditis as they do for infarction. (See Chapter 2 and the preceding discussion on myocardial infarction for details.) Characteristic QRS changes in the precordial leads in pericarditis are absent, a point of difference from infarction.

THE INTRINSIC DEFLECTION OF THE QRS COMPLEX

Because the QRS complex or the depolarization process of the ventricular musculature plays such a significant rôle in interpretation of the

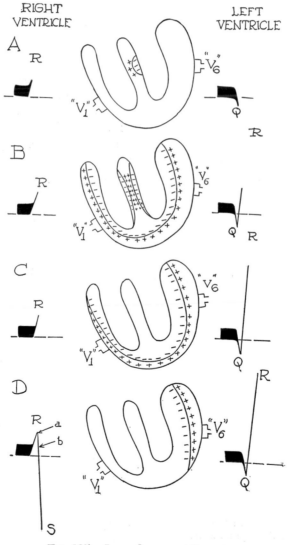

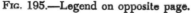

Fig. 195.—Legend on opposite page.

electrocardiogram, it is advisable to give it more thorough consideration, especially with regard to its intrinsic deflection. As indicated by Wilson and his associates, the changes in the QRS complex are usually more permanent than T wave changes and do not, of course, manifest as readily recognizable changes in response to disease states as the T waves.

Definition.—The intrinsic deflection records the instant at which the area of cardiac muscle immediately below a unipolar epicardial electrode has been completely depolarized. It can be seen in figure 195A that when

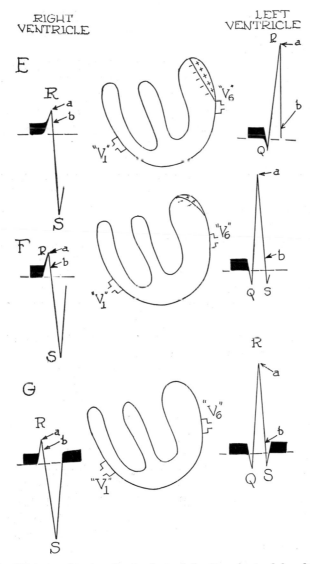

FIG. 195.—Diagram showing the intrinsic deflection obtained by direct unipolar precordial electrodes placed directly on the surface of the right and left ventricles; *a* indicates the beginning of the intrinsic deflection and *b* the end.

a wave of depolarization migrates through the ventricular musculature, the left side of the septum is depolarized first, rendering the electrode over the right ventricle relatively positive and the one over the left ventricle relatively negative. A small R and a small Q wave are consequently recorded by each electrode respectively (Fig. 195A). Within a short time the wave of depolarization is initiated in the subendocardial regions of the right and left ventricles and in the right side of the septum. This reduces the degree of positivity of the electrode upon the surface of the right ventricle and causes the galvanometer string to return toward the isoelectric line. The electrode upon the surface of the left ventricle becomes relatively positive, and the string moves upward or in a positive direction (Fig. 195 B).

Since the wall of the right ventricle is relatively thin, the process of depolarization migrating through that ventricle suddenly arrives at the epicardium under the electrode, while the thicker left ventricular wall is still being depolarized (Fig. 195C). Upon completion of depolarization in the area of muscle immediately under the electrode over the right ventricle, the vector force directed toward the electrode disappears, and an intrinsic deflection, which begins at *a* and ends at *b*, is inscribed (Fig. 195D). The force in the left ventricle, which is still being depolarized, is directed away from the electrode and is unopposed. Thus, the recording over the right ventricle shows a sudden large downward deflection following the intrinsic deflection.

The process of depolarization in the left ventricle continues toward the electrode over that ventricle, the degree of positivity increasing as it approaches the electrode (Fig. 195D). Then the area of muscle immediately under the electrode suddenly becomes depolarized, and the galvanometer string returns to the isoelectric line (Fig. 195E). This sudden downstroke of the R wave is the *intrinsic deflection* for that point over the left ventricle. It begins at *a* and ends at *b* (Fig. 195E), *i.e.*, begins at the peak of the R wave and ends at the isoelectric line.

As the wave of depolarization continues within the free wall of the left ventricle at its base, the electrode on the surface of the left ventricle becomes relatively negative, and an S wave is inscribed (Fig. 195F). With completion of ventricular depolarization the galvanometer string returns to the isoelectric line (Fig. 195G).

It is thus evident that the *intrinsic deflection divides the QRS complex into two parts:* (1) The portion of the QRS which precedes the intrinsic deflection represents electric forces produced by depolarization of cardiac muscle before that in contact with the electrode and (2) that portion of the QRS which follows the intrinsic deflection results from electric forces caused by depolarization of muscle after that in contact with the electrode is depolarized.

Since in clinical studies it is not possible to place an electrode directly upon the surface of the epicardium, *direct precordial electrodes* cannot be used; instead *indirect precordial electrodes* are employed, *i.e.*, electrodes are placed upon the chest near the heart. Although the latter positions are not as satisfactory, they may be suitable for practical clinical purposes and probably record primarily changes in the cardiac muscle immediately under the electrode. Furthermore, because of the use of indirect precordial electrodes the deflection is not a true intrinsic deflection, and it is referred to as the intrinsicoid deflection.

The Intrinsicoid Deflection of the Normal QRS Complex

Certain facts noted by Wilson and associates concerning the intrinsicoid deflection are worth mentioning. Most of these are self-evident.

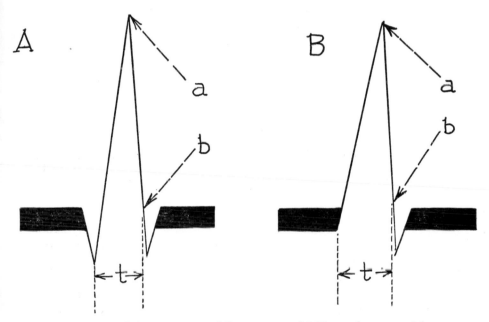

Fig. 196.—*A* and *B* represent two different types of QRS complexes; *a* and *b* represent the beginning and ending of the intrinsicoid deflection, and time *t* denotes roughly the length of time required for the depolarization process to migrate from the subendocardial layer of muscle to the subepicardial layer.

1. Since the intrinsicoid deflection represents a moment, it is **timeless**. For this reason, no electrocardiograph utilized clinically can **record** it accurately.
2. The amplitude of the intrinsicoid deflection represents essentially the difference in potential between the endocardial and epicardial surfaces of the myocardium subjacent to the precordial electrode during depolarization. The height of the deflection is not an index of the thickness or of the degree of hypertrophy of the ventricular wall.

3. The amplitude of the intrinsicoid deflection indicates essentially the degree of the positive potential attained under the precordial electrode.

4. Since the process of depolarization approaches but does not pass the precordial electrode, a negative deflection results from the depolarization processes migrating in a distant muscle and in a direction away from the electrode (Fig. 196). When distant muscle is not depolarized, the intrinsicoid deflection terminates at the isoelectric line (Fig. 197), and a simple R wave is recorded.

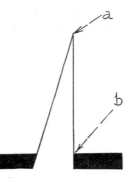

Fig. 197.—An intrinsicoid deflection beginning at *a* and ending at *b*, in which no distant myocardial tissue is depolarized after the muscle immediately under the precordial electrode. The intrinsicoid deflection terminates the QRS complex, and a simple R wave is inscribed.

5. Whenever the intrinsicoid deflection for the left ventricular surface terminates before the QRS ends, the terminus is displaced downward and an S wave follows it; this is explained by the fact that distant muscle is depolarized and the precordial electrode is rendered relatively negative.

6. A septal Q wave indicates a negative cavity and a normal bundle branch on that side.

7. Since the intrinsicoid deflection indicates the instant when the depolarization process reaches the subepicardial layer of muscle, the later it appears in the QRS complex, the thicker the wall of the ventricle must be. This is true for the left ventricle only and provided, of course, conduction of the process of depolarization is normal.

8. It is obvious from Figure 195 and from the foregoing discussion that:
   a. *The intrinsicoid deflection from the precordium of the right ventricle*
      1. Occurs early in the QRS complex.
      2. Is small or low in amplitude.
      3. Is followed by a broad and deep S.

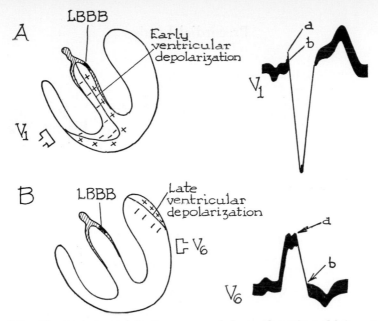

Fig. 198.—The intrinsicoid deflection, as recorded over the right and left ventricles in complete left bundle branch block. It is evident that the intrinsicoid deflection occurs on time in V_1 and late in V_6 and that the slurred, notched, and deformed portion of the QRS complex occurs after the intrinsicoid deflection in V_1 and before it in V_6. Consult the text of Chapter 2 and Chapter 3 for further discussions of the mechanisms of alterations in the process of depolarization in left BBB.

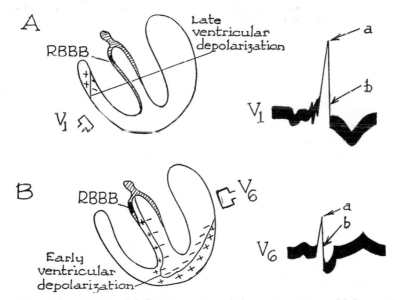

Fig. 199.—The intrinsicoid deflection, as recorded over the right and left ventricles in complete right bundle branch block. It is evident that the intrinsicoid deflection occurs late in V_1 and on time in V_6, and that the slurred, notched, and deformed portions of the QRS occur before the intrinsicoid deflection in V_1 and after it in V_6. Consult the text of Chapter 2 and Chapter 3 for further discussions of the mechanism of alterations in the process of depolarization in right BBB.

13   (103)

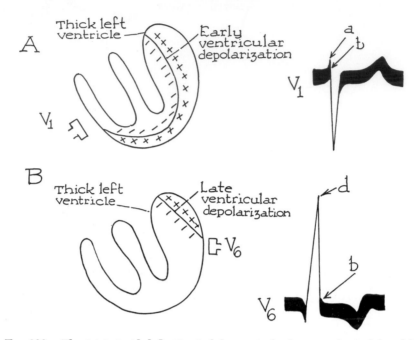

FIG. 200.—The intrinsicoid deflection in left ventricular hypertrophy is delayed because the greater thickness of the ventricular wall increases the time required for the process of depolarization to penetrate the epicardium.

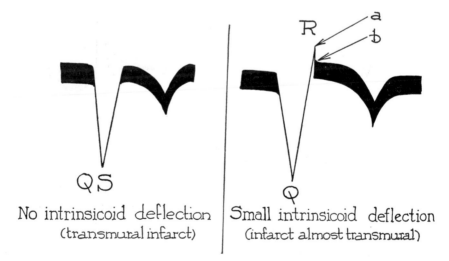

FIG. 201.—The intrinsicoid deflection is altered in myocardial infarction. If the precordial electrode is placed over the infarcted zone and the infarct is *transmural,* the intrinsicoid deflection is abolished; if some viable muscle remains, a small late deflection exists. The mechanisms for these alterations in the intrinsicoid deflection are obvious.

b. *The intrinsicoid deflection from the precordium of the left
   ventricle*
   1. Occurs late in the QRS complex.
   2. Is tall or great in amplitude.
   3. Is followed by a small or no S wave.
   4. Is almost always preceded by a Q wave and an R wave of
      great amplitude.

The Intrinsicoid Deflection and Abnormal QRS Complexes

It is necessary to present only a few examples of the intrinsicoid deflection in abnormal complexes in order to indicate its rôle in the interpretation of such complexes.

1. *Complete Left Bundle Branch Block*
   In complete left BBB the intrinsicoid deflection in V_5 or V_6 is *late*
   (Fig. 198). This is to be expected, since the impulse must travel
   from the right ventricle through the interventricular septum before
   it reaches the Purkinje system of the left side, to be distributed
   to the subendocardial layer of the left ventricular muscle. Consequently, the QRS is wide and the subepicardial layer of muscle on
   the free wall of the left ventricle is depolarized late, delaying the
   intrinsicoid deflection. The latter is preceded by a wide, slurred, and
   notched R wave, and no septal Q wave is present. The intrinsicoid
   deflection in V_1 or V_2 is normal in time or early, for obvious reasons,
   and is followed by a wide, slurred, and notched S wave (Fig. 198).
2. *Complete Right Bundle Branch Block*
   In complete right BBB the intrinsicoid deflection is *late* in V_1 and V_2
   and early or normal in time in V_5 and V_6. In V_1 and V_2 it is preceded by the slurred, notched, and deformed S wave (Fig. 199).
3. *Left Ventricular Hypertrophy*
   In left ventricular hypertrophy the intrinsicoid deflection is *late* in
   V_5 and V_6 (*i.e.*, in a precordial lead recorded over the left ventricle),
   because the depolarization wave must traverse a thick layer of
   wall of muscle before arriving at the subepicardial surface; in V_1
   and V_2, however, it is normal in time (Fig. 200).
4. *Right Ventricular Hypertrophy*
   In right ventricular hypertrophy the intrinsicoid deflection is *late* in
   V_1 and V_2 and normal in time in V_5 and V_6, provided no hypertrophy exists in the left ventricle.
5. *Myocardial Infarction*
   If there is myocardial infarction with transmural infarction, the
   intrinsicoid deflection is abolished in the precordial lead recorded
   with the epicardial electrode over the infarcted zone (Fig. 201). If
   there is little muscle still viable, then a deep Q wave is followed by
   a small R wave and a late, small intrinsicoid deflection.

Chapter 4

DISORDERS OF THE HEART BEAT

THE cardiac arrhythmias constitute a group of cardiac physiologic states characterized by disturbances in the order or rate of depolarization and repolarization. These may or may not be indicative of cardiac disease.

The electrocardiograph is the instrument *par excellence* for the demonstration and diagnosis of disorders of cardiac mechanism. For example, one can frequently determine by clinical methods that the patient has premature beats, but the electrocardiogram will usually indicate their site of origin.

In general, it may be stated that the nerve supply of the heart consists of the *sympathetic* nervous system, which supplies the heart generally, and the *parasympathetic* nervous system, which supplies the SA and AV nodes. The parasympathetic nervous system is limited to the supraventricular regions of the heart. Afferent fibers of the vagus nerve and sympathetic nervous system transmit reflex stimuli from the viscera, lungs, aorta, carotid sinuses, great veins, arteries, coronary vessels and auricles to the cardiovascular centers of the central nervous system. Efferent fibers pass from the cardiovascular centers to the SA and AV nodes, where these impulses produce their effects through the medium of chemical and physical phenomena. Distention of the visceral pleura retards the cardiac rate (Hering-Breuer reflex). Distention of the great veins of the heart accelerates the cardiac rate (Bainbridge reflex). Reflexes such as the Bezold-Jarisch reflex, as well as others originating about the heart, great vessels, and lungs, should be studied for better appreciation of cardiac mechanisms.

The *inherent* control of the cardiac beat results from the ability of the cardiac conduction tissue and musculature to initiate the depolarization process. If the heart is isolated from its nervous control, the SA *node* will initiate the depolarization process at approximately 76 beats per minute. If the SA node is removed, the AV *node* will initiate a rhythm at a rate of about 60 beats per minute. If the AV node is also obliterated, the bundle of His will act as pacemaker and inaugurate impulses at a slower rate, about 50 beats per minute. If the bundle of His is also removed, the ventricular muscle will initiate the depolarization process at a rate of 30 to 40 beats per minute.

In general, impulses pass from the SA node by way of the auricular musculature to the AV node, the bundle of His, the bundle branches, the Purkinje network, and then to the muscle of the ventricle. They may also travel in the reverse direction.

At this point it is wise for the reader to refamiliarize himself with the physiology of the cardiac beat, as such considerations are outside the scope of the present discussion.

NORMAL SINUS RHYTHM

This is the normal cardiac rhythm that occurs in the normal resting subject. The rate varies between 60 and 101 beats per minute in the normal adult. The impulse is regularly initiated at the SA node and passes through the conduction tissue of the heart, as stated in the preceding paragraph (Fig. 202).

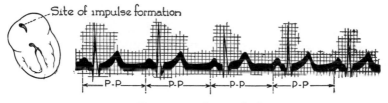

Fɪɢ. 202.—Normal sinus rhythm.

SINUS ARRHYTHMIA

Sinus arrhythmia is a normal rhythm characterized by alternating periods of rapid rate with periods of a slower rate. These changes usually vary with respiration, the periods of rapid rate occurring during the end of inspiration and the periods of slower rate at the termination of expiration (Fig. 203). Such changes may also occur with rhythmic contractions

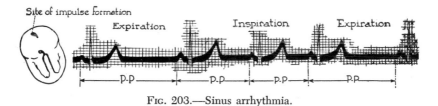

Fɪɢ. 203.—Sinus arrhythmia.

of the spleen or blood vessels and with rhythmic variations in blood pressure.

During the period of rapid rate, the P waves tend to be more peaked and occasionally the P–R interval is somewhat shorter. As sinus arrhythmia is frequently caused by altered activity of the Hering-Breuer reflex from the lung, stretching of the lung causes vagal inhibition of the SA node. It is possible to have sinus arrhythmia manifested in rhythmic changes in rate of the auricles or of the P waves only. This is especially true in atrioventricular block (Fig. 204).

Sinus arrhythmia is most frequently found and most highly developed in young individuals. It has no clinical significance and is more apparent in slowly beating hearts.

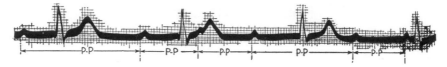

FIG. 204.—Sinus arrhythmia in the presence of complete AV block.

SINUS TACHYCARDIA

Sinus tachycardia is a type of cardiac mechanism in which impulses are liberated at the SA node at a rate greater than 100 beats per minute in adults. In infants a resting rate greater than this is usual. A rate of 100 in an adult is normal sinus rhythm, whereas that of 101 is indicative of

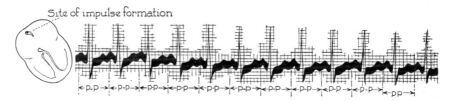

FIG. 205.—Sinus tachycardia. The rate is greater than 100 beats per minute.

sinus tachycardia (Fig. 205). Some laboratories consider a resting rate of more than 90 beats per minute as indicative of sinus tachycardia. Sinus tachycardia, as far as the SA node and atria are concerned, may exist in the presence of a slow ventricular rate, as in complete atrioventricular block. Usually, however, the impulses from the normal pacemaker are conducted through in the normal fashion.

Sinus tachycardia may be associated with thyrotoxicosis, fever, certain emotional disturbances, exercise, or with other states. It may or may not be clinically significant and in itself is not indicative of cardiac disease.

SINUS BRADYCARDIA

Sinus bradycardia is a cardiac mechanism in which impulses originate at the sinus node at a rate of 60 beats per minute or less. The P–R interval tends to be slightly longer than for the usual normal resting rates, and the P waves are somewhat low (Fig. 206).

Sinus bradycardia is not suggestive of cardiac disease. It occurs normally in athletes and other normal persons, as well as in patients with arteriosclerosis, jaundice and certain cerebral abnormalities.

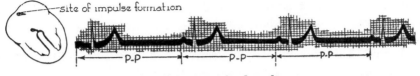

FIG. 206.—Sinus bradycardia.

SINUS ARREST—AURICULAR STANDSTILL—SINOAURICULAR BLOCK

Sinus arrest, auricular standstill, and sinoauricular block present somewhat similar electrocardiographic patterns under certain circumstances.

Sinus arrest is due to temporary failure of the SA node to initiate impulses, usually for a moment only. It occurs in some patients after carotid sinus pressure and is a functional state.

Sinoauricular block occurs as a result of an organic lesion within or surrounding the SA node that produces interference with the transmission of impulses from the node. Such lesions are rare.

Auricular standstill is said to occur whenever an impulse fails to depolarize the auricle and, therefore, an auricular contraction does not take place. This may be due to sinus arrest or to sinoauricular block.

In *sinoauricular block* the electrocardiographic pattern will vary considerably, depending upon the degree of block. If it is complete, failure of a *nodal rhythm or idioventricular rhythm* to develop would prove fatal. In the case of a 2 to 1 block, the electrocardiographic pattern resembles sinus bradycardia. If the block is irregular, a P wave and probably a QRS complex and T wave would be absent when they would ordinarily be expected. There is a true "dropped" beat at such a time, *i.e.,* a whole cardiac cycle drops out (Fig. 207).

Sinus arrest results in failure of the SA node to initiate depolarization of the auricles (Fig. 208). This, or sinoauricular block, may cause sudden death. Sinoauricular block is sometimes caused by quinidine, digitalis or organic cardiac disease. When the SA node temporarily fails to initiate an impulse or when its impulse fails to reach the AV node because a transient lesion completely surrounds the node, one of three things may happen if the heart does not cease beating entirely (Fig. 208).

1. The SA node may resume its activity, and the cardiac beat resumes its normal mechanism (Fig. 208, *1*).

2. The AV node may initiate an impulse (nodal escape, Fig. 208, *2a* and *2b*), and then the SA node takes over from there on, or the AV node may continue as the pacemaker (*nodal rhythm*).

3. Some other portion of the heart, such as the ventricular musculature, may initiate the response (*ventricular escape*, Fig. 208, 3). The SA node usually takes over from there, or the ectopic focus in the ventricle may continue as the pacemaker (*idioventricular rhythm*).

If, after a period of cardiac standstill due to *sinus arrest* or *sinoauricular* block, normal sinus rhythm is resumed, auricular and ventricular depolarization and repolarization occur by impulses traveling over the usual pathways. A P wave with a QRS complex will be seen to follow the pro-

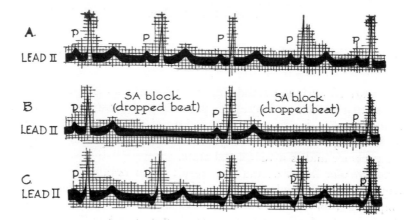

Fig. 207.—*Sinoauricular block*. (*A*) a normal tracing; (*B*) a 2:1 sinoauricular block (the tracing resembles sinus bradycardia); (*C*) complete sinoauricular block with nodal rhythm.

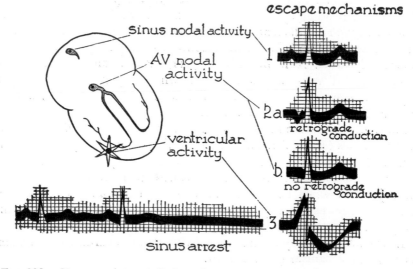

Fig. 208.—Sinus arrest is usually brought on by increased vagal stimulation. The SA node fails to initiate an impulse and, as a result, no auricular or ventricular depolarization occurs. *1, 2* and *3* show the types of mechanisms that may take over the problem of initiating impulses. (See text for details.)

longed period free from any electric activity as recorded by the electro-cardiogram (Fig. 209).

When the AV node initiates the first impulse after the auricular stand-still (*nodal escape*), ventricular depolarization will take place in the usual manner, and a QRS complex similar in configuration to that present before

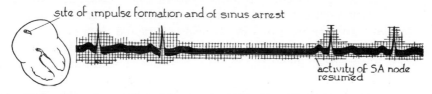

FIG. 209.—*Sinus arrest*, followed by activity of the SA node. The P waves and QRS complexes return to the configuration present before the sinus arrest.

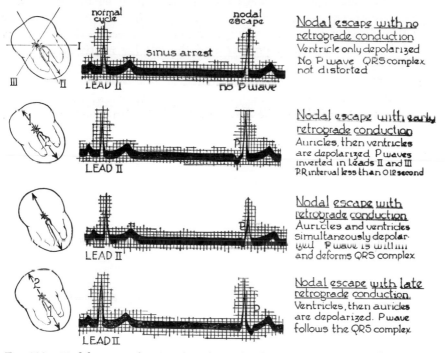

FIG. 210.—Nodal escape, showing the relationship between the QRS complex and the P wave in lead II. (See text for details.)

the sinus arrest will follow the period of no electric activity. Should the impulse from the AV node travel to the auricle, initiating auricular de-polarization in a direction opposite to the usual one (*retrograde conduction*), the P waves will be different in configuration from those recorded prior to the sinus arrest, and the P–R intervals will be shorter than 0.12 second (Fig. 210). The P wave may be found before, within, or after the QRS complex, depending upon the relative times of ventricular and auricular depolarization. The various possibilities for lead II are shown in figure 210. If there is no retrograde conduction, a P wave will not be present. As a rule, the SA node assumes the pacemaker role again after one escape beat is initiated in the AV node.

If the AV node continues to initiate the depolarization processes, *a nodal rhythm* is produced. It has been shown that if an impulse traveled in a direction from the right shoulder to the left iliac crest, an upright deflection would be inscribed in all leads. In nodal rhythm with *retrograde conduction,* the auricular depolarization wave travels from the AV node in a retrograde direction, *i.e.,* in a direction from the left iliac crest toward the right shoulder. Depolarization processes traveling in this direction produce downward deflections in leads II and III. Thus, in electrocardiograms showing nodal rhythm with retrograde conduction, the P waves are inverted in leads II and III. Remember that the *source* or positive charge precedes the wave of depolarization, and the *sink* or negative charge follows it. During retrograde conduction the right arm and left arm are relatively positive and the left leg relatively negative, thus reversing the flow of current through the galvanometer and causing a negative P wave in lead II and lead III.

The P wave in lead I may be inverted, diphasic, or upright, depending upon the exact direction of the auricular depolarization process (Fig. 211).

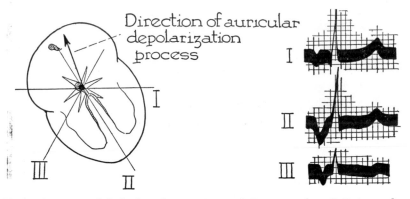

FIG. 211.—AV nodal rhythm showing inverted P waves, short P–R interval, and *normal QRS complexes.* A shallow P wave is present in lead I, and a deep negative wave is present in leads II and III. The P wave may occur before, within, or after the QRS complexes, depending upon the relative time of auricular and ventricular depolarization.°

°Henceforth, in most of the diagrams illustrating an impulse originating from an ectopic focus, the triaxial reference system will be shown with its center at the ectopic site. A heavy arrow beginning at the center of the triaxial reference system and ectopic focus indicates the mean direction of the depolarization process concerned with the abnormal mechanism. From the triaxial reference system and the arrow (a "vector" without proportional magnitude, to use the term vector loosely) it is possible, if perpendicular lines are dropped to the respective lead lines of the triaxial reference system, to learn the direction of the complexes concerned in the completed electrocardiogram.

It is usually low in amplitude in this lead, regardless of its shape. If there is nodal rhythm without retrograde conduction, no P waves are recorded.

If the P wave differs from those originating in the SA node and the P–R interval is greater than 0.12 second, then depolarization was probably initiated in the auricle. This rare phenomenon is spoken of as *auricular escape* (Fig. 212). The shape of the P waves will depend upon upon the site of origin in the auricles. If it is *low in the auricles,* the P waves will have the same configuration as in nodal escape or nodal rhythm with retrograde conduction, except that the P–R interval will usually be greater than 0.12 second.

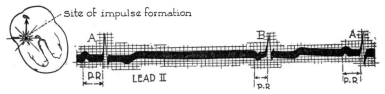

FIG. 212.—*Auricular escape* and low auricular P wave. The P wave at B is different from that at A. The P–R interval is greater than 0.12 second at B but less than the normal P–R interval represented at A.

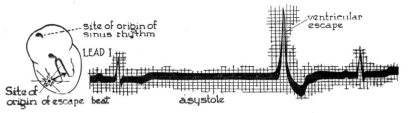

FIG. 213.—*Ventricular escape* with the SA node resuming the rôle of pacemaker.

Ventricular escape: In the event that the SA node, AV node, or auricle fails to initiate the impulse, the ventricular musculature itself, possibly as a result of the accumulation of metabolites, will initiate depolarization of the ventricles (*ventricular escape*). As the direction and course of the depolarization process are abnormal, so the QRS complex will be abnormal, being notched, slurred, and wide and having the appearance of ventricular premature beats (Fig. 213). As a rule, the SA node immediately resumes its function as pacemaker of the heart. Should the ectopic focus in the ventricle continue to act as pacemaker, as is likely to occur in complete *sinoauricular block,* the phenomenon is referred to as *idioventricular rhythm.* If there is retrograde conduction with ventricular escape or idioventricular rhythm, a P wave of the type described for nodal escape with retrograde conduction will occur within the QRS complexes or T waves. Obviously, these P waves are often difficult to identify.

PREMATURE BEATS—ECTOPIC BEATS—EXTRASYSTOLES

Although these three terms are sometimes used more or less synonymously, certain differences exist.

A *premature beat* is a beat which occurs earlier than would be expected in the basic rhythm. This term is preferred over the other two.

An *ectopic beat* is one originating outside of the usual site of impulse formation, which is thought to be located in the "head" of the SA node. Thus, an ectopic beat may originate in the "tail" of the SA node, in the auricle, in the ventricle or elsewhere than the head of the SA node. Ectopic beats are not necessarily premature, since they include beats arising from the AV node or ventricle, as in nodal rhythm or idioventricular rhythm. Escaped beats are ectopic but not necessarily premature.

Extrasystoles are extra beats which are sandwiched in between two other beats of the basic mechanism. The interpolated premature ventricular beat is an example of a true extrasystole.

There are three main types of *premature beats:* (1) *auricular,* (2) *nodal or junctional* (AV node), and (3) *ventricular.*

AURICULAR PREMATURE BEATS

Auricular premature beats may arise in the SA node or, more commonly, in the auricular musculature. The interval between the premature auricular contraction and the preceding normal beat is shorter than the interval between two beats of the basic mechanism. A P wave is *always present* in auricular premature contractions, although it may be difficult to identify in some leads. The P wave may be diphasic, isoelectric or inverted in any lead. If the depolarization process originates in the SA node, the P wave will be shaped like those of the basic rhythm in the same lead. The compensatory pause is *incomplete* in auricular premature beats, *i.e.,* the sum of the P–P intervals of the impulses before and after the premature beat is *less than* the sum of two consecutive P–P intervals of the basic rhythm (Fig. 214).

If the *auricular impulse arises low in the auricle,* the depolarization process will travel for the most part from the low site in the auricle in a retrograde fashion toward the SA node. In such an instance the P wave will be isoelectric, diphasic, upright or inverted and usually of low amplitude in lead I and negative in leads II and III. The P–R interval will usually be greater than 0.12 second (Fig. 215). It is obvious that if the site of origin of the impulse is low in the auricle but far from the AV node, the P–R interval may be somewhat increased. The P–R interval is sometimes long if the premature beat is extremely early and begins early in the refractory period of the auricle, before it has fully recuperated from the preceding contraction.

The compensatory pause is incomplete in auricular premature beats, as the ectopic focus in the auricular muscle initiates a wave of auricular depolarization that travels to the SA node and discharges its impulse before the impulse in the node is fully developed. The SA node then re-establishes impulses at its original rhythm.

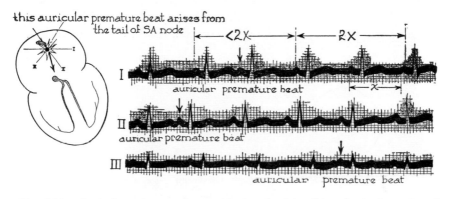

Fig. 214.—*Auricular premature beats* with site of origin of impulse in the region of the tail of the SA node. The P waves of the premature contractions are normal in appearance and they have the appearance of the P waves of the basic rhythm. The QRS complexes are similar to the QRS complexes of the basic mechanism. The compensatory pause is incomplete. ($< 2X$ = interval of time measured from the P wave of the normal cycle just before to the P wave of the normal cycle just after the premature contraction. X = interval of time between the P waves of two successive normal cycles of the basic mechanism.)

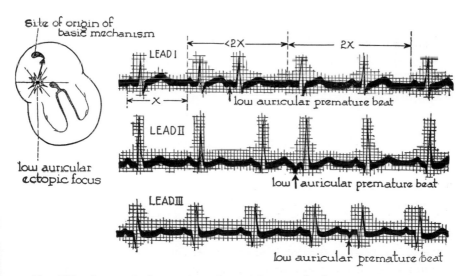

Fig. 215.—*Low auricular premature beats*. The auricular beat is premature in time, the P–R interval is usually greater than 0.12 second, and the P waves are inverted in lead II and lead III. The compensatory pause is incomplete.

AURICULAR PREMATURE BEATS WITH ABERRATION

In the preceding discussion of premature beats it was stated that the QRS complexes following the premature auricular contractions are similar to the QRS complexes of the basic mechanism in the same lead. If the auricular premature beat comes at a time when the bundle branches or ventricular musculature are partially refractory, abnormalities (slurring, notching and widening) of the QRS complex result, due to disturbances

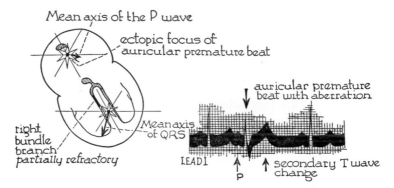

Fig. 216.—*Auricular premature beat with aberration.* Wide, slurred QRS complexes and secondary T wave changes are produced by the inequality in the refractory state of the two bundle branches. The P wave is abnormal in configuration, since auricular depolarization arose from an abnormal site.

in the order of ventricular depolarization. At times the duration of the QRS complex is greater than 0.10 second (Fig. 216). Widening may be particularly apparent. As a result of the QRS changes there are sometimes *secondary T wave changes.* Such a wide complex with altered T waves may resemble a ventricular premature beat on casual inspection.

BLOCKED PREMATURE AURICULAR BEATS

Blocked premature auricular beats occur when an early auricular premature beat is initiated but cannot be transmitted through the AV node, due to its complete refractory state. The electrocardiographic picture of this condition is characterized by an abnormal P wave which is not followed by a QRS complex. This resembles heart block except that the P wave of the premature beat is abnormal in configuration, indicating an abnormal site of impulse formation. The P wave is premature in time. The configuration of the P wave will, of course, vary with the site of its origin (Fig. 217).

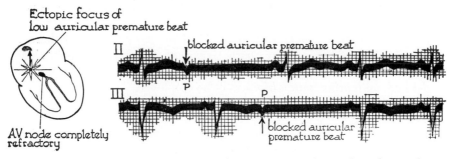

FIG. 217.—*Blocked premature auricular beats* originating from a focus low in the auricles. The abnormal P waves are not followed by QRS complexes.

MULTIPLE AURICULAR PREMATURE BEATS

Two or more auricular premature beats occurring in succession are indicative of this condition.

MULTIFOCAL AURICULAR PREMATURE BEATS

This diagnosis is made whenever there are two or more auricular premature beats *in the same lead* in which the *P waves of the premature contractions are of different form,* indicating that they have originated from different foci in the auricles.

NODAL (JUNCTIONAL) PREMATURE BEATS

Premature contractions which originate from the AV node are called *nodal or junctional premature contractions* and are characterized by the presence of a P wave if there is retrograde conduction into the auricles. The P waves are of abnormal shape (Fig. 218) and may occur before, within, or after the QRS complex (Fig. 210). There is a P–R interval of less than 0.12 second if the P wave precedes the QRS complex. The QRS complexes are only deformed when the P waves fall within the QRS complexes or when the nodal premature beats occur sufficiently early to reach the ventricular muscle or conduction tissue during the refractory period with resultant aberration (Fig. 218). *As a general rule, the QRS complexes are similar in configuration to those of the basic mechanism.*

If there is retrograde conduction, the P waves are of variable configuration in lead I but of low amplitude and inverted in leads II and III, for the reasons discussed previously for nodal escape with retrograde conduction (Fig. 211).

The compensatory pause may be incomplete if there is retrograde conduction and if the depolarization process in the auricles initiated at the AV node discharges the impulse in the process of formation in the SA node. If there is no retrograde conduction, the compensatory pause will be complete (Fig. 219).

When *conduction is defective in the Purkinje system,* so that there is alteration of the QRS complex characteristic of arborization block, along with other characteristics of nodal premature beats, the term *premature nodal beat with arborization block* may be employed.

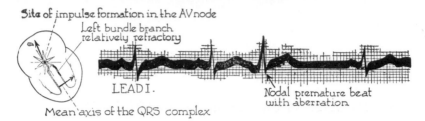

Fig. 218.—*Premature nodal beat with aberration.* Ventricular depolarization precedes auricular depolarization. The QRS complex is wide and slurred because of disturbances in the order of ventricular depolarization.

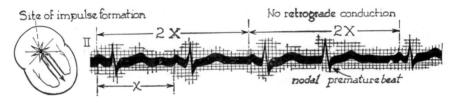

Fig. 219.—The compensatory pause is complete when there is no retrograde conduction with *nodal premature contractions.*

If there are nodal premature contractions without retrograde conduction, a P wave is not found in close association with the premature beat unless, due to the impulse initiated at the expected time in the SA node, the P wave happens to occur at about the time that the QRS complex of the nodal premature beat is inscribed. In the absence of retrograde conduction, the SA node continues with its basic rhythm, and auricular depolarization waves (P waves) will occur "on time." The configuration of the QRS complexes in the absence of retrograde conduction will have the same characteristics as described previously for nodal premature beats with retrograde conduction.

Obviously, nodal premature contractions may be multiple, but electrocardiographically they are *never multifocal.*

VENTRICULAR PREMATURE BEATS

When a premature contraction originates from a focus in one of the two ventricles, it is called a *ventricular premature contraction.* It has the following characteristics:

1. **The** QRS complex is *distinctly abnormal, being wide, slurred, and notched.*

2. *The compensatory pause is complete.*

3. *The P wave resulting from an impulse initiated by the SA node occurs at the expected time and may or may not be discernible* in the deformed QRS complex. The T wave is usually opposite in direction to the main deflection of the QRS complex (Fig. 220). This constitutes a *secondary T wave change.*

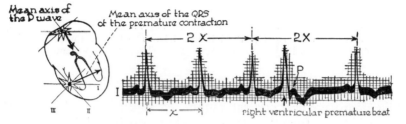

Fig. 220.—*Right ventricular premature beat,* showing the high, wide QRS complex with secondary T wave change. The P wave is visible in the abnormal complexes and falls at the expected time. The compensatory pause is complete. (2X = the interval of time measured from the normal QRS complexes before and after the abnormal QRS complex, and X = the interval of time between two successive normal QRS complexes of the basic mechanism.) Obviously, in the presence of auricular fibrillation or the like, rules for the compensatory pause do not apply.

The compensatory pause is complete, since the ventricular ectopic depolarization process does not disturb the basic rhythmic activity of the SA node.

In certain instances *retrograde conduction* may occur. The depolarization process, which starts in the ventricles, travels through them into the auricles. The SA node may be discharged early, and the compensatory pause will be incomplete. Retrograde conduction may be recognized on the electrocardiogram, since the *abnormal QRS complex* is associated with *inverted P waves in leads II and III.*

Right Ventricular Premature Contractions

If the ectopic focus is in the *right ventricle,* the depolarization process travels from the right ventricle of the heart through the interventricular septum to the left ventricle. The course of the impulse, initiated in the ectopic focus in the right ventricle, follows a course that is comparable in many respects to LBBB (see Chapter 2). The mean electric axis then is running toward the positive electrode, LA electrode, of the lead I axis of the triaxial reference system. Therefore, the main deflection (one of greatest duration) of the QRS complex is up or positive in lead I. It is usually extremely slurred, notched, and deformed in many ways (Fig. 221).

14

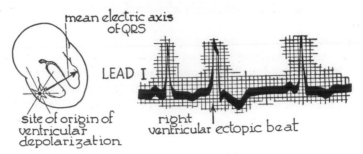

FIG. 221.—*Right ventricular premature beat.* The mean electric axis of the QRS complex travels from the right to the left ventricle. The QRS complex is wide and notched and *positive* in lead I. Secondary T wave changes are present.

Left Ventricular Premature Contractions

If the premature beat originates in the *left ventricle,* the depolarization process will travel from the left to the right ventricle and the *main deflection* (one of greatest duration and most deformed) *of the QRS complex is down or negative* in lead I (Fig. 222). The course of the impulse through the ventricle is similar to that in right BBB (see Chapter 2).

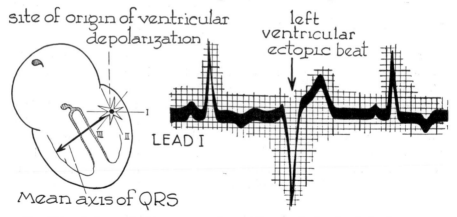

FIG. 222.—*Left ventricular premature beat.* The ventricular depolarization process travels from the left ventricle toward the right ventricle producing mainly a downward deflection in lead I. The configuration in lead I may be constructed from the complexes of the premature beat by means of Einthoven's equation ($QRS_1 = QRS_2 - QRS_3$). The main deflection of the QRS complex is *negative* in *lead I.*

The premature contraction of ventricular origin *must be recorded in lead I* in order to determine the ventricle from which it originated. Lead II and lead III are of no value in determining whether a ventricular premature contraction was initiated in the right or left ventricle. The *precordial leads* indicate, as in BBB, the site of origin of a ventricular premature contraction. The reasons for this are essentially the same as those presented for the diagnostic use of precordial leads in BBB.

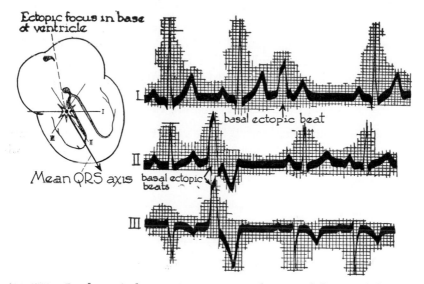

FIG. 223.—*Basal ventricular ectopic contraction*. The major deflection of the QRS complex is upright in *all three standard leads*.

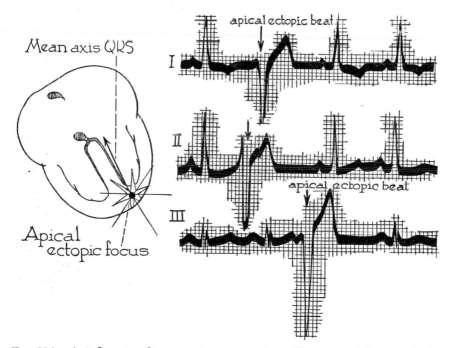

FIG. 224.—*Apical ventricular premature contraction*. The major deflections of the QRS complexes are down in *all three standard leads*.

Basal Ventricular Premature Contractions

If the ectopic focus is in the base of the ventricles, the impulse travels from the base toward the apex of the heart, and the major deflections (ones of greatest duration and usually most deformed) of the QRS complexes are upright in *all three standard leads* (Fig. 223).

Apical Ventricular Premature Contractions

If the ectopic ventricular focus is in the *apex*, the impulse travels toward the base, and the major deflections (ones of greatest duration and usually most deformed. of the QRS complexes are down in *all three standard leads* (Fig. 224).

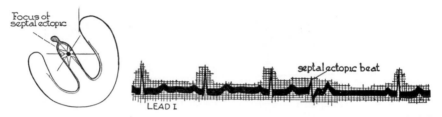

FIG. 225.—*Septal ventricular premature contraction.* The QRS complex is only slightly deformed and there are usually some secondary T wave changes.

Septal Ventricular Premature Contractions

In the case of *a septal ventricular premature beat,* a focus somewhere in the septum initiates the depolarization process. Spreading more or less equally in all directions, it reaches the Purkinje system of both ventricles quickly and more or less simultaneously. The depolarization impulse reaches the musculature of both ventricles about the same time as it would were the origin in the SA node. For that reason, the QRS complex is not much wider than for the normal basic mechanism. Once the impulse reaches the Purkinje system, it is distributed throughout the ventricles in a more or less normal fashion. Thus, at first glance, the QRS complex appears normal in itself, although closer inspection reveals it to be of slightly different configuration from the QRS complexes of the basic mechanism and it is not early enough to be altered by aberration. The auricular rhythm is not disturbed; the auricular depolarization wave (P), therefore, falls at the usual time, within, or shortly after, the QRS complexes of the septal ectopic beat (Fig. 225). Other characteristics of a ventricular premature contraction are usually present.

Multiple Ventricular Premature Contractions

Multiple ventricular premature beats are identified by the occurrence of at least two ventricular premature beats in succession.

Multifocal Ventricular Premature Contractions

Multifocal ventricular premature contractions are present when there exist in *any one lead* at least two ventricular premature beats which are definitely of different configuration, therefore, have arisen from different foci in the heart (Fig. 226). This rule does not apply unless the QRS complexes of the premature contractions, which have different configurations, are present in a *single lead,* regardless of which lead it is, or the premature beats recorded in different leads can be proved to originate from different foci by application of Einthoven's law.

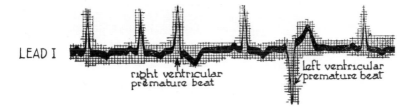

LEAD I

right ventricular premature beat

left ventricular premature beat

Fig. 226.—*Multifocal ventricular premature contractions.* The first is of right ventricular origin and the second of left ventricular origin.

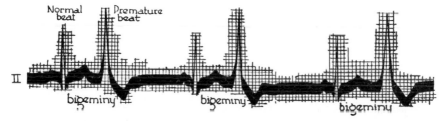

Normal beat

Premature beat

II

bigeminy

bigeminy

bigeminy

Fig. 227.—*Bigeminy.* A normal beat is followed by a premature beat, which in this instance is of ventricular origin. This is known as coupling.

BIGEMINY AND TRIGEMINY

Bigeminy is a term applied to the grouping in pairs of arterial pulse beats. This may be produced by: (1) a premature contraction following every normal contraction (coupling), the compensatory pause and prematurity accounting for the grouping effect (Fig. 227); or (2) the presence of an AV block of every third auricular impulse, so that two normal ventricular complexes (QRS) are followed by complete absence of one QRS complex.

Trigeminy is a term applied to the grouping of arterial pulse beats in *threes.* This may be produced by: (1) a premature contraction that regularly follows every two normal beats, or (2) two successive premature contractions following a normal beat, the compensatory pause accounting for the grouping effect (Fig. 228). Of course, as far as the pulse is concerned, the premature contraction must be of sufficient strength to produce a pulse wave. The grouping of the cardiac cycles into threes in such a manner, when detected by auscultation of the heart or by electrocardiography, is termed *trigeminy*. Trigeminy may also be produced by (3) a complete AV block of every fourth impulse that reaches it from the auricles.

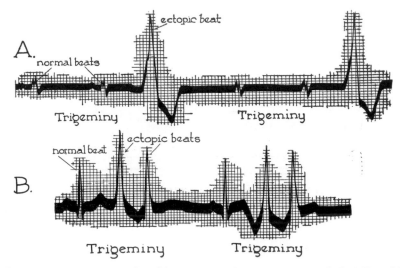

FIG. 228.—*Trigeminy* produced by two normal contractions regularly followed by a ventricular premature beat (*A*), or one normal contraction followed by two ventricular premature beats (*B*).

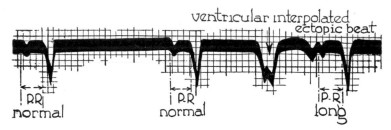

FIG. 229.—*Interpolated ventricular extrasystole.* The period of the cardiac cycle containing the interpolated premature beat is prolonged over that of the basic mechanism, and that following the premature beat is shortened slightly. Since the auricular cycle is unaffected, the change in length of the cardiac cycle is due to variation in length of the P–R intervals.

INTERPOLATED PREMATURE BEATS

An interpolated premature beat is one that is "sandwiched" between two normal contractions. The latter occur more or less "on time" (Fig. 229). The cycle containing the premature beat is disturbed, being somewhat lengthened, whereas the cycle following it is shortened. The P–R interval following the ectopic beat is prolonged, due to the relative refractory state of the conduction tissue.

COMBINATION COMPLEXES

Combination complexes may be of two types: (1) *auricular* and (2) *ventricular.*

(1) *Auricular combination complexes:* If an AV nodal premature contraction with retrograde conduction should occur rather late, so that the depolarization wave of the auricle initiated by the SA node is already under way, two simultaneous depolarization processes within the auricles would be responsible for the inscription of the P wave. The P wave of the completed record shows the influences of the two depolarization processes and is called an *auricular combination complex.* The P–R interval is short and, of course, the P wave is deformed (Fig. 230).

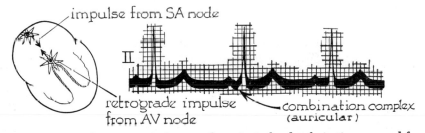

Fig. 230.—*Combination auricular complex.* Auricular depolarization occurred from an impulse originating in the SA node and from an impulse by retrograde conduction from the AV node.

Impulses may be discharged simultaneously from the two sites of their origin to produce auricular depolarization simultaneously in every instance, or one may begin first and the other follow soon after. This can result in extreme diversity of P wave configurations.

Auricular combination complexes are particularly likely to occur when the cardiac mechanism is in transition from an SA to an AV nodal rhythm.

(2) *Ventricular combination complexes* may be produced when a ventricular premature contraction occurs so late that auricular depolarization initiated by the SA node is already under way. This may cause the first part of the QRS complex to be abnormal or similar to the first part of a QRS complex of ventricular depolarization initiated from the same ectopic focus recorded in the same lead. This QRS complex starts like the other QRS complexes produced by the same ectopic focus, but before the ventricular depolarization has been under way very long, the impulse from auricular depolarization passes through the AV node and enters the Purkinje system to complete depolarization of the ventricles in a normal

fashion. This results in a terminal portion of the QRS complex with configurations more or less similar to the basic QRS complexes of the same lead produced by the normal sinus mechanism. The resultant QRS complex is a *combination complex*. It is produced by a depolarization process initiated from an ectopic focus in the ventricle and completed by the normal impulse initiated in the SA node or *vice versa*. The P–R interval is short or absent (Fig. 231).

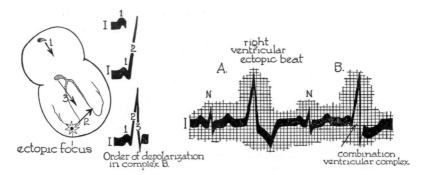

Fig. 231.—A combination complex, *B*, due to a late right ventricular premature beat occurring just at the completion of depolarization of the auricles. The combination QRS complex is due to depolarization of the ventricles by an impulse originating from an ectopic focus in the ventricles and an impulse originating from the auricles above, the former initiating ventricular depolarization and the latter completing it. The numerals indicate the orders of depolarization chronologically. Note that the first part of the combination complex *B* is similar in configuration to the first part of the right ventricular premature beat *A*, and the terminal portion of complex *B* resembles the terminal portion of the normal complexes, *N*.

SIGNIFICANCE OF PREMATURE BEATS

Though more common in the presence of cardiac disease, premature beats may *occur normally* in persons without any disease of the heart. In general, they tend to disappear with exercise. If not numerous, multiple auricular or ventricular premature beats are not indicative of cardiac disease. Frequent multifocal ventricular beats are strongly suggestive of myocardial disease. They may precede auricular or ventricular fibrillation or flutter. Premature beats are found associated with infectious states, rheumatic heart disease, thyrotoxicosis, arteriosclerotic heart disease or any type of organic as well as functional cardiac states.

PARASYSTOLE

Parasystole is a mechanism resulting from the *rhythmic initiation of impulses from two foci in the heart:* (1) the SA node and (2) an ectopic focus in the auricles, the usual site; ventricles; or any other site in the heart. The site of impulse formation which initiates impulses at the most rapid rate controls the basic rhythm of the heart, is the *"pacemaker,"* and expresses itself as such in the completed electrocardiogram. The *superimposed rhythm,* produced by the site of less rapid impulse formation, is not manifested at that moment on the completed electrocardiogram. For example, if the SA node initiates impulses at the rate of 80 beats per minute and an ectopic auricular focus inaugurates impulses at the rate of 60 beats per minute, the basic rhythm will be controlled by the SA node. If the sinus rhythm is reduced to less than 60 beats per minute by respiration, rest, or carotid sinus pressure, the ectopic focus in the auricles will then be responsible for the basic rhythm and will act as the pacemaker. The *parasystolic focus* (the focus in the ectopic site) *is recognized by the essentially absolute regularity of its impulse formation,* that is, the cycle lengths do not usually vary by more than 0.01 second from each other. The *constancy* of the rhythm of the ectopic pacemaker, *i.e.,* usually to within 0.01 second, may be stated as follows: The interval in

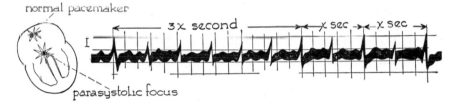

FIG. 232.—*Parasystole.* There is rhythmic initiation of impulses from two foci in the heart. One is the normal pacemaker in the SA node, which initiates impulses at a normal rate with sinus arrhythmia and is shown to the left of the figure. The parasystolic focus is in the AV node, which initiates impulses at a slower but *absolutely regular* rate. The initiation of impulses occurs simultaneously by both foci but the impulses initiated by the parasystolic focus are only manifested in the electrocardiogram when the myocardium is not refractory. The time interval in seconds between any two complexes initiated by the parasystolic focus has a common divisor that yields a whole number for a quotient.

seconds between any two complexes produced by the ectopic pacemaker, no matter how far apart, will be divisible by a common denominator that always results in a whole number as a quotient. In fact, this test is usually applied to confirm the existence of a parsystolic rhythm. Although many of the parasystolic impulses are blocked by the refractory state of the muscle and are not manifested on the electrocardiogram, careful measurement of the complexes arising from this focus demonstrates its absolute rhythmicity. Impulses from the SA node, however, vary considerably from cycle to cycle with respiration, splenic contraction, and other factors (Fig. 232). Parasystole has the same significance as premature contractions. It may be added that some observers are dubious of the existence of parasystole.

PAROXYSMAL TACHYCARDIA

Paroxysmal tachycardia is a cardiac mechanism initiated by an ectopic focus or possibly a circus movement in the heart, in which there is a rapid succession of impulses occurring with absolute regularity of rhythm for seconds, minutes, hours, or days. There are *three* types of paroxysmal tachycardia named for the site of the ectopic focus in the heart initiating the impulses: (1) *auricular*, (2) *nodal*, and (3) *ventricular*.

Paroxysmal tachycardia is said to be produced by an *ectopic focus* in the auricle, AV node, or ventricle. There are some who believe that a *circus movement* under special circumstances may be responsible for the mechanism. The circuit in auricular tachycardia, similar to that in flutter, is thought to be into and out of the SA node and into and out of the AV node in the case of nodal tachycardia. Auricular and nodal tachycardia may be terminated by *carotid sinus pressure*, since the AV and SA nodes are richly supplied by vagus nerve endings. Carotid sinus pressure is usually not effective in relieving ventricular paroxysmal tachycardia; these attacks sometimes terminate spontaneously. This is thought to be due to an accidental increase in vagus tone, the sensitivity of which is heightened by greater hydrogen ion content of the cells, as occurs with fatigue following prolonged periods of tachycardia.

The essential characteristics of *all types* of paroxysmal tachycardia are:

1. They begin suddenly, *i.e.*, within a space of one beat.

2. The first beat is a premature beat.

3. The beats are absolutely regular, *i.e.*, the cycles usually do not vary from each other by more than 0.01 second. Gradual changes in the cycle length, due to changes in rate, do occur when the tachycardia persists for long periods of time. Ventricular tachycardia tends to be somewhat more irregular.

4. If and when the paroxysm ceases, its termination occurs suddenly, usually within the interval of one or two beats.

5. Carotid sinus pressure usually has one of two effects. It either does not affect the tachycardia at all or it stops or changes its rate suddenly and completely. An increase in vagus tone may be brought about by pressing on the eyeball (the oculocardiac reflex) with the same results.

6. The disturbances, of course, occur in paroxysms. Either the attack is terminated within a matter of minutes, hours, or days, or congestive heart failure develops and death ensues. With prolonged tachycardia there is a decrease in cardiac output, blood pressure, pulse pressure, pulse volume and diastolic filling of the coronary arteries and flow, with a resultant *coronary type of pain*. Gangrene and signs of disturbances within the central nervous system occasionally occur. The cardiac rates, both auricular and nodal, tend to range between 140 and 240, usually around 160 beats per minute. Rates as high as 300 have been recorded, particularly in infants.

Auricular Paroxysmal Tachycardia

Auricular paroxysmal tachycardia presents the electrocardiographic characteristics of a rapidly regular, repeated series of auricular premature beats. The P waves may not be easily identified, but when discernible, they are seen to be of abnormal form, as they are usually produced by a focus in the auricular muscle outside the normal pacemaker or SA node (Fig. 233). Consult the discussions on auricular premature beats for the reasons for changes in configuration of P waves. The shape and character of the P wave depend upon the site of origin of the depolarization

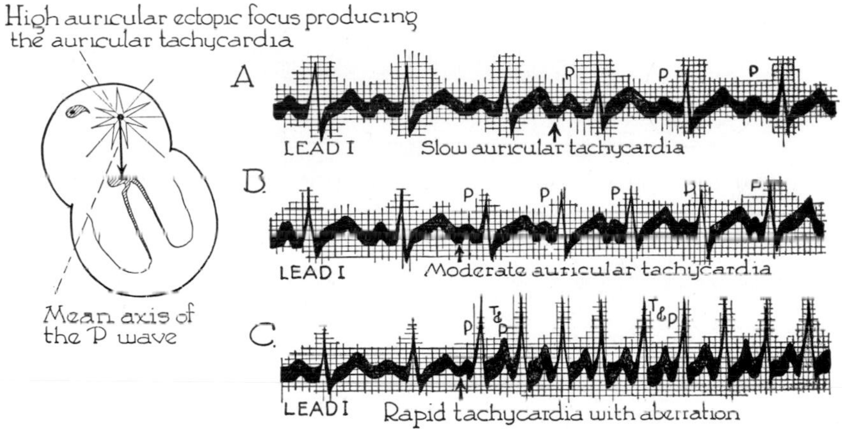

Fig. 233.—*Paroxysmal auricular tachycardia.* The beginning and end of the paroxysms are abrupt. Cycle lengths do not vary more than 0.01 sec. A, Rate is 90 beats per minute. P waves visible on descending limb of T wave. C, Rate is 220 beats per minute, and P waves cannot be identified. This cannot be differentiated with certainty from nodal tachycardia. It is best designated as *supraventricular paroxysmal tachycardia.* Extreme aberration due to defective ventricular depolarization because of defective intraventricular conduction may occur. The arrows indicate the beginning of the period of tachycardia, which continues throughout the remainder of the tracing.

process in the auricle. For example, if the site is low in the auricles, the P waves will be inverted in leads II and III. (See Auricular Premature Beats, page 204.) If the tachycardia is prolonged, relative ischemia with primary T wave changes develops. This may also result in defective intraventricular conduction with changes in the QRS complexes characterized by slurring, notching, and widening (Fig. 233).

Nodal (Junctional) Paroxysmal Tachycardia

Junctional (nodal) paroxysmal tachycardia resembles auricular tachycardia in all respects except that the P waves are inverted in leads II and III if there is retrograde conduction (Fig. 234) or are entirely absent if there is no retrograde conduction. (See Nodal Premature Beats.) Often it is impossible to differentiate nodal from auricular tachycardia when the rate is rapid, and the presence or absence of the P waves cannot be determined. In such instances, the term *supraventricular tachycardia* is applied. The *clinical significance* of auricular and nodal paroxysmal tachycardia is essentially the same as that of auricular and nodal premature beats. They do not indicate disease of the myocardium. If they persist at a rapid rate, congestive failure may result, but the myocardium returns to normal after the paroxysm stops.

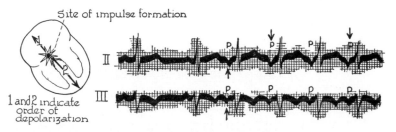

FIG. 234.—*Nodal paroxysmal tachycardia* with retrograde conduction. The P waves are inverted in leads II and III. The arrows indicate the beginning of the tachycardia.

Paroxysmal Ventricular Tachycardia

Paroxysmal ventricular tachycardia is produced by an ectopic focus in the ventricles initiating impuses at a rapid, regular rate (Fig. 235). It is strongly suggestive of cardiac disease in patients in whom it is not precipitated by administration of digitalis and related drugs, quinidine, or

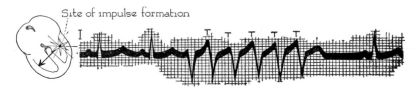

FIG. 235.—*Ventricular paroxysmal tachycardia.* The paroxysm starts and stops abruptly. Although each individual QRS complex of the abnormal mechanisms closely resembles the other, they do vary to some slight extent. Rate is rapid. The rhythm may not be as regular as in supraventricular tachycardia. P waves occur at the regular times but are only recognized occasionally.

other drugs. It sometimes precedes ventricular fibrillation, which may be the terminal event, or it may occur after coronary occlusion or in other severe organic cardiac disease. It does not respond to carotid sinus pressure or to vagal stimulation.

Paroxysmal ventricular tachycardia presents the following characteristics:

1. The auricular rate is not disturbed unless there is retrograde conduction. The P waves, which occur at regular intervals, can sometimes be identified in the bizarre complexes. If the result of retrograde conduction, they are of abnormal form.

2. The QRS complexes are wide, slurred, sometimes variable in appearance, and regular in rhythm. They have the same characteristics as those described for ventricular premature contractions. (See discussions on page 208.)

It may be said that the terms *paroxysmal ventricular tachycardia, ventricular tachycardia, and paroxysmal ventricular flutter* are more or less synonymous. If *paroxysmal ventricular tachycardia* and *ventricular flutter* are physiologically dissimilar, the differences are not demonstrable electrocardiographically.

AURICULOVENTRICULAR BLOCK

Auriculoventricular block may be classified as follows:
1. *Incomplete or partial AV block.*
   A. Incomplete AV block without dropped ventricular beats (QRS complexes), prolonged AV conduction time only.
   B. Incomplete AV block with dropped ventricular beats. When the P–R interval varies, showing progressive lengthening until an impulse from the auricle is completely blocked at the AV node, a dropped ventricular beat, the mechanism is referred to as the *Wenckebach phenomenon.* The block *may occur at regular intervals,* such as a conduction of every other impulse to the ventricles, there being two auricular complexes (P waves) to one ventricular complex (QRS). This is known as 2:1 AV block. Various degrees of block, such as 3:1, 4:1, and so forth, may occur.
2. *Complete AV block, i.e.,* no impulses pass through the AV node.
   A. The ventricular pacemaker may be located in the bundle of His below the lesion in the AV node responsible for the block, producing QRS complexes similar to those seen in nodal rhythm.
   B. The ventricular pacemaker may be located in the *ventricular musculature* (idioventricular rhythm), in which case the QRS complexes are wide, slurred, and notched and have the characteristics of ventricular premature beats. The *ventricular pacemaker may shift from time to time* from one site to another within the ventricles.

Incomplete Auriculoventricular Block

Incomplete or partial AV block is due to functional or organic inhibition of the transmission of the impulses from the SA node and auricles through the AV node. The inhibiting process may be within the auricular muscle or in the AV node itself.

In its mildest form there is merely *slight lengthening of the P–R interval* without "dropped" ventricular complexes (Figs. 85 and 86). In general, a P–R interval greater than 0.20 second in patients with cardiac rates over 70 beats per minute indicates the presence of *incomplete AV block*. At slower rates the upper limit of normal is 0.21 second. This disorder constitutes *definite evidence of myocardial disease.*

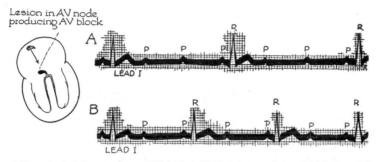

Fig. 236.—*A*, 3:1 incomplete AV block. *B*, 2:1 incomplete AV block. When the auricular impulses are blocked at the AV node, there is absence of QRS complexes following the P waves.

In its more severe form there is *periodic dropping* of the *ventricular complex,* which produces variations in the ratios of the number of auricular to ventricular complexes. If there are 4 auricular complexes to 3 ventricular complexes, one dropped ventricular complex (QRS) occurring for every 4 auricular complexes (P waves), the block is referred to as 4:3 incomplete or partial AV block. More serious states of block are 2:1, 3:1, 4:1 (Fig. 236).

When the P–R interval increases progressively until a QRS complex fails to follow the P wave and this process repeats itself successively, the mechanism is known as the Wenckebach phenomenon. This has already been discussed in Chapter 2 (Fig. 86).

Complete Auriculoventricular Block

Complete AV block is usually due to organic discontinuity of the conduction tissue in the AV node or bundle of His, producing individual and unrelated activity of the auricles and the ventricles. Since the auricular impulses fail to pass through the AV node, an ectopic focus in the ventricles usually becomes the pacemaker of the ventricles, *i.e.,* an *idioventricular rhythm* is established as a compensatory mechanism to keep the patient alive. The SA node continues to initiate depolarization processes in the auricles at a relatively rapid or normal rate, while the ventricles are rhythmically depolarized by impulses initiated at the ectopic site at a rate about half as rapid as that of auricular depolarization. The P waves are of normal configuration but the QRS complexes are deformed, the nature of the deformity depending upon the site of formation in the ventricles.

Variations in the configuration of the QRS complexes obey the characteristics described for ventricular premature beats. If the ventricular depolarization process originates in the *junctional tissue* (bundle of His) just below the lesion in the AV node, the QRS complexes are of relatively normal appearance (Fig. 237A). The ventricular rate is usually about 50 beats per minute.

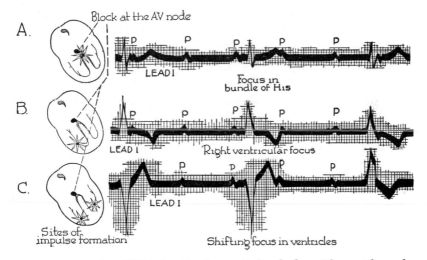

Fig. 237.—*Complete AV block with idioventricular rhythm.* The auricles and ventricles are beating independently of each other. In all three examples, A, B, and C, the auricular rate is 76 beats per minute. A, The junctional tissue (bundle of His) below the lesion in the AV node is acting as a pacemaker and is producing ventricular complexes of relatively normal form at a rate of about 50 beats per minute. B, The idioventricular rhythm is produced by a focus in the right ventricle. QRS complexes are wide and notched and occur regularly about 30 times per minute. C, The idioventricular rhythm is produced by a shifting pacemaker in the ventricles. The first two complexes are from the left ventricle, the third from the right ventricle.

If ventricular depolarization is initiated in the *right* or *left ventricle,* the ventricular complexes will be abnormal, resembling right or left ventricular premature beats (Fig. 237B and C).

If there is a *shifting pacemaker in the ventricles,* that is, if ventricular depolarization is initiated by impulses liberated by various ectopic foci in the ventricles, the ventricular complexes will be variable in appearance (Fig. 237C). The rhythm maintained by a ventricular ectopic focus is known as *idioventricular rhythm.*

The following electrocardiographic characteristics of complete AV block are definite and simple to detect if a tracing of sufficient length is available:

1. The auricular rate is usually about twice the ventricular rate. This is evidenced by about twice as many P waves as QRS complexes per unit of time.

2. The P–R intervals are extremely variable; few, if any two, possess the same length. In fact, there are no true P–R intervals, since the auricular impulses are not conducted to the ventricles.

3. The auricles and ventricles beat independently of each other as evidenced by the two foregoing findings. Any relation of a P wave to a QRS complex is, therefore, a "hit and miss" occurrence.

4. An idioventricular rhythm is present.

The presence of any type of AV block is *definite evidence of cardiac disease*. Complete AV block indicates a serious cardiac state, especially if due to organic disease. Complete and incomplete block may be due to congenital defects in the conduction tissue, particularly in association with interventricular septal defects, or to arteriosclerotic disease of the coronaries, syphilitic cardiac dsease, or any type of organic cardiac abnormality. Incomplete, and even complete, AV block are frequently produced by many infectious diseases, such as rheumatic fever and diphtheria. It is sometimes caused by toxic doses of digitalis, in which case it is particularly reversible.

INTERFERENCE DISSOCIATION

Interference dissociation is a disturbance in cardiac mechanism usually produced by toxic amounts of digitalis. It resembles complete AV block in its general appearance. Digitalis causes the auricles to contract at a

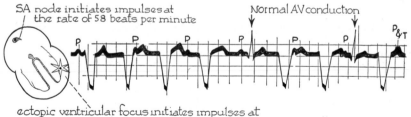

Fig. 238.—*Interference dissociation*. The ventricular rate is 80 and the auricular rate is 58 beats per minute. The auricles and ventricles are beating independently. At the arrow normal conduction through the AV node occurred and the P, QRS and T waves are normal in appearance. These complexes also have, on casual inspection, the appearance of premature contractions. The idioventricular rhythm is initiated by an ectopic focus in the left ventricle.

relatively *slow* rate, and the ventricles, because of a nodal rhythm, or idioventricular rhythm, contract at a *more rapid rate*. Since there is no retrograde conduction, the auricles respond to the impulses initiated at the SA node. The ventricles, on the other hand, can respond to the impulse from the auricles only if they are not in a state of refraction when they reach the AV node or ventricles. Should the impulses reach the AV node and ventricles when they are in a responsive state, a QRS complex that *seems premature* in time is inscribed. There is, therefore, independent beating of the auricles and ventricles, with occasional normal conduction of impulses throughout. This state, *interference dissociation,* should never be confused with complete AV block since: (1) in the former the *auricular rate is less* than the ventricular rate, whereas in the latter the reverse is true, and (2) in the former there will be *occasional* instances of normal conduction (Fig. 238). The mechanism returns to normal with cessation of digitalis therapy and elimination of the drug from the body.

ELECTRIC ALTERNATION

Electric alternation is a cardiac mechanism in which the electrocardiographic pattern consists of alternation of the form and amplitude of the QRS complexes and T waves. Every other QRS complex is of similar

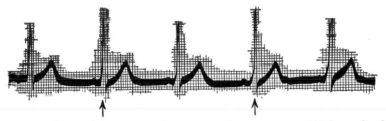

Fig. 239.—*Electric alternation.* Alternate R and T waves are of high amplitude, as shown by the arrows. The alternate waves are similar in configuration but different in amplitude from the other alternate waves.

form and amplitude, two successive complexes being of different forms and amplitudes (Fig. 239). The alternation may affect some or all of the waves of the cycle. Electric alternation is occasionally associated with clinical alternation in the force of the arterial pulsation (*pulsus alternans*).

Electric alternation may be due to a 2:1 partial cardiac block located at some site in the ventricles. Alternate impulses penetrate the barrier, whereas the others pass around it. It has been stated that alternation results usually when only half of the heart is depolarized on alternate beats (*pulsus alternans*). This state sometimes occurs in normal hearts beating at rapid rates for long periods of time or in mild digitalis intoxication. It occurs, of course, in diseased hearts even when the heart is beating slowly. Sometimes it is produced by a prolonged refractory period in certain portions of the diseased heart.

Electric alternation has the same *significance* as the cardiac mechanism producing it; when associated with tachycardia or digitalis intoxication, it has little importance; when associated with pulsus alternans, organic cardiac disease, and a slow rate, the prognosis is grave.

15

CARDIAC MECHANISMS PRODUCED BY CIRCUS MOVEMENTS
OR RELATED PHYSIOLOGIC PHENOMENA

The reader should acquaint himself with the physiologic concepts of *circus movements*. Without a knowledge of these, it is impossible to learn intelligently the electrocardiographic manifestations of *fibrillation* and *flutter*. It is well to know how they initiate waves of depolarization, the relationship of their onset to the refractory period of the myocardium, the influence of an electric stimulus on the mechanism, the relation of circus movements to paroxysmal tachycardia, as well as many other phases of the problem. Recent textbooks of physiology, the recent studies of C. J. Wiggers and his associates, and the studies of Sir Thomas Lewis and his associates should be consulted especially. It will be assumed in the discussions to follow that the reader has a thorough knowledge of circus movements.

Auricular Fibrillation

Auricular fibrillation is a cardiac mechanism produced by rapid irregular depolarization of the auricles with an irregular response of the ventricles to certain impulses from the auricles which penetrate the AV node.

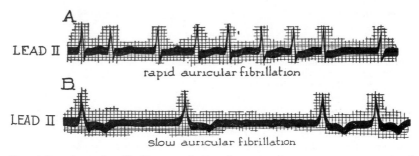

FIG. 240.—*Auricular fibrillation.* A, Rapid ventricular response or rate; B, slow ventricular response or rate. The P waves are absent, and the QRS complexes are absolutely irregular in occurrence. The form of the QRS complexes, especially the amplitudes, vary somewhat. The fibrillation waves, irregular variations in the iso-electric line, may be seen in part B of the figure.

Fibrillation is most probably due to: (1) a circus movement which varies in its course from circuit to circuit; (2) variations in the degree of refractoriness of many islands of auricular musculature, *i.e.*, relatively refractory or nonrefractory at the time; (3) many simultaneously active circus movements; or (4) combinations of all these factors. These factors are responsible for the irregularity of the mechanism. The rate of the auricular response varies between 400 and 550 per minute. The AV node is able to respond and to transmit only one out of every 3 or 4 auricular responses, so that the ventricular rate is usually slightly over 100 beats per minute.

In the electrocardiogram, *auricular fibrillation is recognized by the absence of P waves and the irregular inscription of ventricular complexes which vary somewhat in form,* depending upon the amount of aberration resulting from the relative refractory state of the ventricular conduction system or musculature (Fig. 240). Definite P waves are absent because there are many depolarization processes migrating in many directions and, therefore, neutralizing each other electrically, resulting in little to no difference in electric potential from one part of the auricle to the other. Since there is really a *minute difference* in electric potential, close examination of the base line will reveal that it does vibrate slightly and irregularly. For practical purposes, however, it is free from P waves. The small, irregular vibratory waves are sometimes called *fibrillation waves.* Fibrillation may be rapid or slow. When the ventricular response is slow, the absolute irregularity of the QRS complexes is more easily demonstrated.

Exercise in patients with auricular fibrillation increases the rate and irregularity of the ventricular response, in contrast to the disappearance of premature beats on exercise.

Digitalis depresses the conductivity of the AV node, so that the ventricular response to the rapid bombardment by auricular impulses is lessened, with a tendency for the AV node to respond only to the strong impulses reaching it. This slowing in the ventricular rate accounts in large part for the increase in the force of the ventricular contractions, the reduction in pulse deficit and improvement in the patient. The heart beats more efficiently at the slower rate.

Carotid sinus pressure decreases the ventricular rate by depressing AV nodal contraction but does not stop the mechanism as it does in patients with auricular or nodal tachycardia. Pressure on the carotid sinus does not produce auricular standstill as it may in patients with auricular flutter.

Auricular Flutter

Auricular flutter is considered by some to be due to a single circus movement coursing around the orifices of the superior and inferior venæ cavæ and producing a circular path of auricular depolarization. This tends to result in auricular depolarization perpendicular to the lead I line and relatively parallel with the leads II and III lines. *The flutter (f waves), or P waves, are thus seen best* in leads II and III (Fig. 241). The ventricles may respond to every circuit of auricular depolarization (1:1 rhythm) or more frequently to every 2, 3, or 4 circuits, thus producing a 2:1, 3:1, or 4:1 rhythm or block. The relatively long refractory period of the AV node produces the incomplete AV block. The ventricular rate therefore usually varies between 75 and 100 beats per minute, as the auricular rates vary between 200 and 380. It may even exceed 400 beats per minute in infants. Recent experimental studies suggest a single focus as a possible origin of the impulse of flutter, but the data are not convincing enough to discard the concept of the circus movement. Regardless of the mechanism, the electrocardiographic pattern is characteristic.

The electrocardiographic characteristics are as follows:

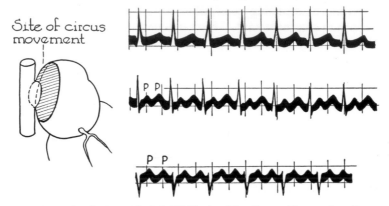

FIG. 241.—Auricular flutter with 2:1 AV block. The flutter (f waves) or P waves are best seen in leads II and III.

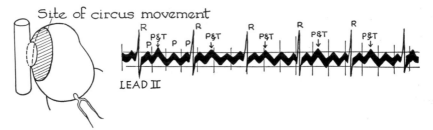

FIG. 242.—*Auricular flutter.* There is a 4:1 AV block. The P waves have a "sawtooth" appearance.

1. The P waves are absolutely regular in rhythm. They are characterized by a rapid upstroke and a more gradual downstroke and by the absence of any isoelectric interval between the waves, reflecting the constant activity of the circus movement (Fig. 242).

2. The ventricular rhythm is regular unless there is a variable AV block. If the AV block changes rapidly, the clinical picture of the mechanism will simulate auricular fibrillation.

3. Carotid sinus pressure causes extreme slowing or standstill of the ventricles by depressing AV nodal contraction so that a functional block occurs, but auricular activity is little affected. Release of the pressure results in reestablishment of the previous rhythm. Following slowing of the ventricles by carotid sinus pressure, the ventricular rate tends to be

irregular for several seconds, due to a variable degree of A–V block, before the previous rhythm is established.

Some observers believe that when the circus movement enters the SA or AV node, it produces paroxysmal auricular or junctional tachycardia. The mechanism is diagnosed as paroxysmal tachycardia and not flutter.

Digitalis often converts flutter to fibrillation, and with cessation of its administration normal rhythm may resume.

Impure Flutter

Occasionally, during a paroxysm of flutter, the P waves may vary slightly from an absolutely regular *rhythm*. At the same time they tend to vary slightly in *contour*. The rhythm of the QRS complexes is usually irregular. The mechanism, therefore, tends to vary between flutter and fibrillation and is referred to as *impure flutter* (Fig. 243) if only slightly different from flutter, or *flutter-fibrillation* if it approaches flutter at one moment and fibrillation at another.

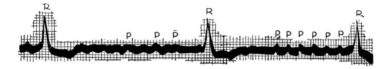

FIG. 243.—*Impure flutter.* The auricular and ventricular complexes vary in form and rhythm, but the mechanism closely simulates auricular flutter.

Ventricular Fibrillation

Ventricular fibrillation is usually not seen electrocardiographically, since it occurs as a terminal event, the patient dying before a recording can be obtained. Paroxysms are occasionally recorded in a dying patient. They are often accompanied by syncope, a type of Stokes-Adams syndrome. The electrocardiogram exhibits irregular, high, wide deflections or QRS complexes (Fig. 244).

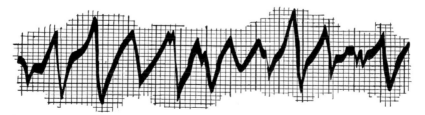

FIG. 244.—*Ventricular fibrillation.* There is absolute irregularity and extreme deformity of the QRS complexes.

Ventricular Flutter

This has already been referred to as *paroxysmal ventricular tachycardia*.

COMBINED MECHANISMS

It is apparent that any two or more of the mechanisms described in this chapter may occur simultaneously. Thus, there may be nodal rhythm and ventricular premature beats, or auricular fibrillation and ventricular premature beats, or sinus arrhythmia and BBB, sinus tachycardia with complete AV block, and so forth.

Chapter 5

CLINICAL APPLICATIONS OF THE
ELECTROCARDIOGRAM

SUGGESTED METHOD OF READING AN
ELECTROCARDIOGRAM

In order to avoid any errors in interpretation of an electrocardiogram, it is necessary that a definite, organized plan of study of the record be followed. The following approach is suggested:

1. The tracing should be studied to determine first if it is *suitable for reading*. Errors in technic should be excluded.
2. The following measurements should then be made routinely:
    (*a*) Auricular rate.
    (*b*) Ventricular rate.
    (*c*) P–R interval.
    (*d*) QRS interval.
    (*e*) Q–T interval.
3. The *electric axis of the QRS* should be measured in degrees.
4. The *cardiac mechanisms* should be indicated.
    (*a*) The *basic mechanism*, such as sinus tachycardia, normal sinus rhythm, auricular fibrillation.
    (*b*) The *superimposed mechanism*, such as premature contractions, sinus arrest.
5. The various waves and intervals in all leads should be *described*. Mention only *significant* changes that will influence your interpretation, such as a negative T in lead I or a negative T in lead V_6.
6. The significance of the record should be *interpreted*. There usually are *four possible diagnoses*. (Criteria are presented in Lists I, II and III of the Appendix):
    (*a*) The electrocardiogram is *normal*.
    (*b*) The electrocardiogram is *slightly suggestive* of myocardial disease.
    (*c*) The electrocardiogram is *strongly suggestive* of myocardial disease.
    (*d*) The electrocardiogram presents *definite evidence* of myocardial disease.
7. *Remarks* should then be made. Pertinent remarks about the electrocardiogram that have clinical significance may be recorded, such as: " It is *typical* of left ventricular hypertrophy." "It is

compatible with mitral stenosis." "It is compatible with acute peri-carditis." "It is typical of acute anterior infarction." "The T wave changes may be due to digitalis." Requests may be made for chest leads, an electrocardiogram after exercise, or a repeated electro-cardiogram, as deemed necessary.

Remember to be objective when interpreting an electrocardiogram. Adhere to criteria. Allow the physician who is seeing the patient to weigh clinical data and correlate them with the electrocardiographic observa-tions. It is desirable to have at hand as much clinical data as possible during interpretation of the electrocardiogram. The age, sex, weight, build of the patient, and previous medication or procedures should always be available.

The terminology and expressions employed in categories 6 and 7 are admittedly vague. These are probably as satisfactory as any with our present concepts of electrocardiography. They do express the existence of certain cardiac states that have clinical significance. When it is possible to be more definite, by the use of more exact terminology, it is advisable to do so. Such interpretive remarks are expected of the car-diologist or interpreter of the electrocardiogram by most clinicians. It is unfortunate when the physician, who does the clinical workup, is incapable of reading his patient's electrocardiogram. One of the difficul-ties in the application of electrocardiography is the religious acceptance by the patient's physician of an electrocardiographic interpretation made by another, whose reading is often erroneously made without a knowl-edge of the entire clinical picture.

THE ELECTROCARDIOGRAM IN CARDIAC DISEASE

It is impossible in a compendium of this sort to list the numerous elec-trocardiographic patterns encountered in the various types of cardiac disease. Most abnormal patterns are not characteristic of any etiologic type of cardiac disease but are only indicative of myocardial damage, expressed in disturbances in the orders of depolarization and repolariza-tion. Furthermore, most systemic diseases and many normal physiologic states are associated with electrocardiographic abnormalities. There have been many descriptions of the electrocardiogram in systemic diseases, suggesting that it has diagnostic significance, but such claims have not always been supported by the experience of others. From correlation of a knowledge of *anatomy, physiology, pharmacology, pathology* and *elec-trocardiography*, it is possible in most instances to predict, and certainly to understand, the electrocardiogram in *cardiac disease* and in systemic disease.

The student should think in terms of *anatomy, physiology,* and *pathol-ogy.* He should be able to visualize the pathologic and physiologic changes in the heart from the electrocardiogram and *vice versa,* especially if all clinical data are available. For example, if an electrocardiogram presents a long P–R interval, defective intraventricular conduction, a long Q–T interval, and a negative T wave in lead I, he should at once think of a pathologic process producing *diffuse myocardial change.* Both the orders of depolarization and repolarization are disturbed. The lesion has involved the AV node or bundle of His. If the electrocardiogram shows an absent R wave, elevation of the S–T segment, and a negative T wave of the Pardee type in lead V_4, he should think of a *localized area of myocardial infarction* with a central area of dead muscle, a shell of injury, and a shell of ischemia in the anterior portion of the heart immediately under the area of the chest where the precordial electrode was placed. This may be due to a stab wound of the heart, to metastatic carcinoma of the myocardium, or to an embolus or thrombosis of the anterior descending branch of the left coronary artery, and its cause must be determined by the other clinical data. Obviously, if one thinks in terms of *anatomy, physiology* and *pathology,* it then becomes *possible to predict, with a great deal of accuracy, the type of electrocardiogram one would expect in any disease state.*

Serial electrocardiograms are of great importance in the study of cardiac disease. In *acute rheumatic myocarditis,* daily electrocardiograms may show rapid changes as the intensity of the inflammation of the heart increases or decreases. There may be evidence of diffuse myocardial change as the inflammatory process involves the auricles, ventricles, and conduction system with resultant changes in the P wave, the QRS complex, the T wave, and the P–R and the Q–T intervals (Fig. 245).

If the *acute inflammatory process* involves mainly the epicardium, the pattern of *acute pericarditis,* with elevation of the S–T segments in leads I, II and the precordial leads placed over the area of inflammation, will be seen (Figs. 140 and 194).

If an Aschoff nodule develops in the AV node, complete or incomplete *auriculoventricular block* may result (Figs. 170 and 236).

In *chronic rheumatic endocarditis,* the electrocardiographic pattern varies with the valves involved. If the *mitral valve is sclerosed* and *stenosed,* an extra load is placed upon the left auricle and right ventricle. This often results in auricular fibrillation (Fig. 240). The increased left auricular pressure extends to the right ventricle, and the pattern of right axis deviation or right ventricular hypertrophy appears. If the disease is sufficient to injure the right bundle branch, right BBB appears (page 89). The increased pressure may exert its effect on the right auricle, and as a result of right and/or left auricular dilatation and hypertrophy, the P waves become high, wide, and/or notched (Figs. 79 and 246).

If the *aortic valve is sclerosed* and stenosed by the rheumatic process, an extra load is placed on the left ventricle, as it must work against an increased resistance to blood flow. Left ventricular hypertrophy develops (see page 136), and injury to the conduction system may result in left BBB (Fig. 97).

If *both aortic stenosis and mitral stenosis exist simultaneously*, there may be a normal position of the mean electric axis of the QRS complex, as the electric forces responsible for the right and left axis deviations pro-

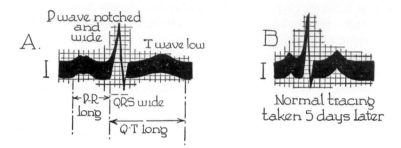

FIG. 245.—*Acute rheumatic myocarditis*, showing signs of diffuse myocardial change. (See text for explanation.) Tracings A and B taken five days apart. Tracing B is normal, probably due to improvement in the inflammatory process.

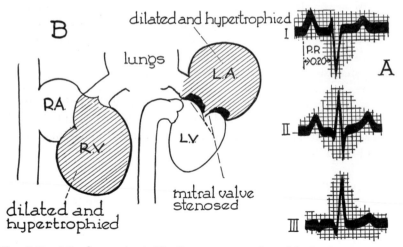

FIG. 246.—*Mitral stenosis.* A, The P waves are wide and high, the P–R interval is prolonged, the QRS complexes are slightly wide and slurred, and there is extreme right axis deviation. B, This diagrammatic sketch shows the chambers of the heart that become dilated and hypertrophied if the mitral valve is sclerosed. Shaded chambers are the ones most diseased.

duced by the individual valvular lesions tend to neutralize each other (Fig. 247).

If, for example, the patient has *congenital pulmonary stenosis*, the increased pressure in the right ventricle, and later the increased pressure in the right auricle, would produce hypertrophy and dilatation of these chambers. As a result, there would first be the electrocardiographic pattern of right axis deviation followed later by primary T wave changes. Because of dilatation, hypertrophy, and disease of the right auricle, the P waves would be large and perhaps peaked or slurred. The T waves in lead I would tend to be inverted, a secondary T wave change. Primary T wave changes may also occur (Fig. 248).

If the patient had *patent ductus arteriosus,* blood would flow from the aorta through the patent ductus into the pulmonary artery. The elevated pressure and blood volume in the pulmonary circulation increase the load on the right ventricle and tend to produce right axis deviation and primary T wave changes. The left ventricle contracts with greater force, in an effort to maintain the systemic blood flow. The left ventricle is working under a disturbance in hemodynamics comparable to aortic re-

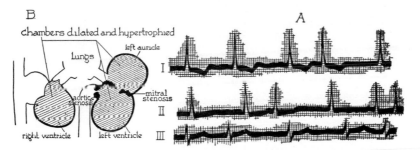

FIG. 247.—*Mitral stenosis and aortic stenosis due to rheumatic fever.* A, There is auricular fibrillation due to strain on the auricles. The QRS axis is normal, as the hypertrophy of the right ventricle as well as that of the left produced by the combined valvular lesions neutralize each other. The QRS complexes are slurred and widened, due to defective intraventricular conduction. There is rightward deviation of the electric axis of the T waves, indicating abnormal repolarization of the ventricles. B, The left auricle, right ventricle and left ventricle are hypertrophied and dilated.

gurgitation or arteriovenous aneurysm; the cardiac output may be three or four times greater than normal. This results in left ventricular hypertrophy with its characteristic electrocardiographic pattern (page 136). The net result of the entire load on the two ventricles is usually no abnormal deviation of the mean electric axis of the QRS complex. Because of the arteriovenous fistula, the systolic pressure is elevated and the diastolic pressure is lowered. As the coronary blood flow decreases with the reduced diastolic pressure, diffuse myocardial change occurs, with production of changes in the P wave, QRS complex, and T wave, and with prolongation of the P–R and Q–T intervals. Such changes are, of course, not diagnostic of the congenital lesion but certainly are indicative of serious myocardial damage (Fig. 249). If right or left ventricular hypertrophy predominates, right or left axis deviation, respectively, may be present.

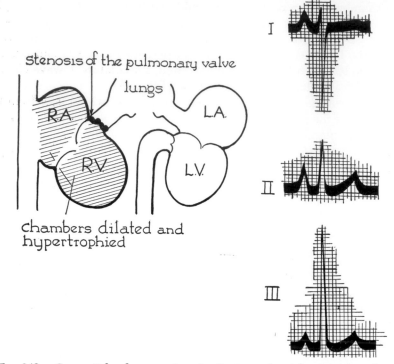

FIG. 248.—*Congenital pulmonary stenosis.* Strain on the right ventricle and auricle produces dilatation and hypertrophy of the right ventricle and auricle, with development of right axis deviation, high, slurred, and wide P waves, and slight prolongation of the P–R interval. The abnormal T waves follow the myocardial damage with *resultant* disturbances in the order of repolarization.

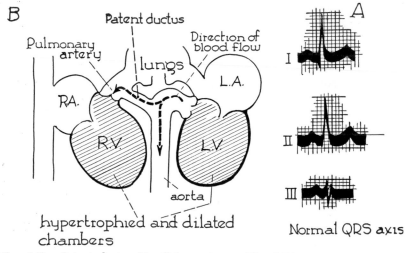

FIG. 249.—*Patent ductus (Botallo) arteriosus.* The QRS axis in this instance is normal. There is evidence of diffuse myocardial change. (See text for explanation.) *B,* The effect of the patent ductus on the heart is shown diagrammatically.

Obviously, from the few examples presented, once anatomic, physiologic and pathologic data concerning any disease state of the heart are correlated with an understanding of the fundamental principles of electrocardiography, the associated electrocardiographic pattern is *relatively simple* to predict and appreciate. It would be absurd to attempt to list all the clinical states with the various possible electrocardiographic patterns, since they are almost unlimited in number, especially when one considers the time-to-time variations, the various stages of the disease processes, and the presence or absence of therapy. The reader should study the subject well enough to be able to draw or predict the electrocardiographic patterns. The many available articles and textbooks on electrocardiography should be consulted for details in specific types of cardiac disease.

Many, if not *all, disease states* influence the electric activity of the myocardium. The recognizable changes are usually limited to disturbances in the order of *repolarization,* evidenced by slight or definitely abnormal changes in the *T waves.* The disease states or even normal physiologic processes that produce abnormal T wave changes, such as an *inversion* of the T wave in lead I, are too numerous to list. Among causes of inversion of T_1 are: drinking of ice water, smoking, syncope, postural syncope, anoxia, endocrine disturbances of many sorts, acidosis, insulin shock, pneumonia or any severe systemic infection, any type of organic cardiac disease, rapid persistent tachycardia, and any organic disease state that produces constitutional effects. Obviously, the *same factors* produce *low, diphasic, or isoelectric T waves,* for a T wave must pass through such configurations before it can change from positive to negative. Many of these changes are purely temporary, whereas others are permanent, depending upon whether or not the etiologic factor is reversible. Streptococcic tonsillitis is an example of the former, and arteriosclerosis illustrates the latter.

Furthermore, such electrocardiographic changes are obviously not characteristic of any etiologic agent and are of no prognostic significance. One may conclude only that at the time of the electrocardiographic recording the repolarization process occurred in an *abnormal fashion.* Only the other clinical data will indicate the prognostic or *clinical significance* of the T wave changes. These T wave changes indicate myocardial disease at the time of the recording. If they are due to *drinking of ice water, smoking,* or *digitalis,* they are reversible and of *no significance;* if they may be due to *essential hypertension, aortic regurgitation,* or *mitral stenosis,* they are irreversible and *extremely significant,* being indicative of serious myocardial disease.

The electrocardiogram without all the clinical data is rarely of great value.

A cardiac study without an electrocardiogram is not complete or thorough.

Not infrequently, the electrocardiogram will indicate the presence of cardiac disease when the entire clinical study is otherwise normal.

CHANGES IN THE INITIAL PORTIONS OF THE QRS COMPLEXES OF THE STANDARD LEADS PRODUCED BY MYOCARDIAL INFARCTION LOCATED IN VARIOUS REGIONS OF THE MYOCARDIUM

Because of the importance of electrocardiography in myocardial infarction, the present discussion is included for completeness. Changes in the S–T segments and in the T waves have already been described in patients with myocardial infarction (page 115). In the following paragraphs the significance of the changes in the initial portions of the QRS complexes in the standard leads will be pointed out. The changes in the QRS com-

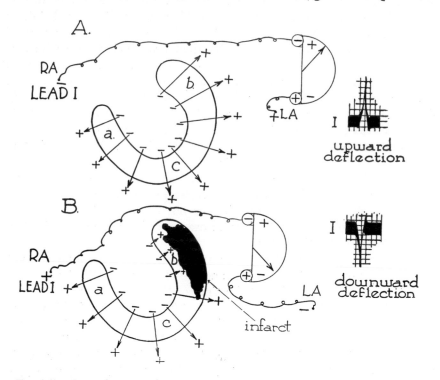

Fig. 250.—In *A*, forces produced by the right and left ventricles are conducted in opposite directions (*a* and *b*). The forces produced by the left ventricle are somewhat greater because of the greater thickness of the left ventricular wall. This is illustrated by the longer arrows at *b*. The forces at the apex (*c*) are unopposed, as there are no forces produced by the open portion of the ventricles at the base. It is simple from the discussion in Chapter 1 to visualize the resultant influence upon the electrodes of the standard leads. In *B*, the infarct in the left ventricle reduces the forces of depolarization there, so that those forces in the right ventricle are now greatest; therefore, there is mainly a negative deflection (Q wave) in lead I.

plexes in the precordial leads have been discussed in Chapter 3. It was indicated previously, and will be explained more clearly, that without the changes in the QRS complexes the changes in the S–T segments and T waves would be of little diagnostic assistance in myocardial infarction.

Because of the death of a localized area of muscle in infarction, the thickness of the wall that is depolarized is reduced. The opposite, uninvolved wall now exerts an electromotive force of depolarization that is unopposed by a similar force in the infarcted wall. In fact, the force in the infarcted wall is completely absent in a transmural infarct. This causes the normal wall to exert a greater influence upon the QRS complex in the completed electrocardiogram (Fig. 250). At this point the reader should reacquaint himself with the nature of the forces and electric fields presented previously in Chapter 2. The action of the two opposing forces might be more vividly illustrated by two horses of about equal strength pulling against each other. If one of the horses were suddenly killed, the equilibrium of forces would be suddenly upset, and the force exerted by the living horse would predominate. Not only will infarction alter the amount of electric potential offered by the opposite walls, but also the position of the electrodes will influence the resultant QRS complexes in the completed electrocardiogram. The QRS complexes in leads I, II, III and in the chest leads (Chapter 3) should, therefore, be correlated to form characteristic electrocardiographic patterns determined by the location of the infarct. These different patterns make it possible to localize myocardial infarction sharply. Some of the prominent patterns of infarction follow.

Posterior Myocardial Infarction

The portion of the heart involved in posterior infarction is the posterodiaphragmatic area of the left ventricle and adjacent portion of the septum. This area is ordinarily nourished by the branches of the right coronary artery. Such an infarct produces an $R_1Q_2Q_3$ pattern for the initial portion of the QRS complexes in the standard leads (Fig. 252). Changes in the precordial leads are discussed on page 175.

It may be recalled that if the electrocardiogram is analyzed as in determining the vectorcardiogram shown on page 62, a *QRS E-loop* (henceforth referred to simply as the QRS loop) is formed by graphing several of the innumerable instantaneous axes (Fig. 65) that constitute the mean electric axis of the entire QRS complex (Fig. 63). This QRS loop may be used as an aid in the analysis of the electrocardiogram in the same manner as the mean electric axes are used. However, with the QRS loop, any instantaneous axis may be chosen, from which a corresponding portion of the QRS complex can be reproduced. The *initial* instantaneous axis of the QRS loop is selected for a study of the QRS patterns in infarction. The loop aids in determining the *initial* QRS changes that take place in myocardial infarction.

As indicated on page 250, the QRS loop can be studied more accurately when recorded by means of a cathode ray oscilloscope to produce the spatial vectorcardiogram. However, such apparatus is not available to every physician. He can secure crude, but satisfactory, data by obtaining the initial portions of the QRS loop from the three standard limb leads.

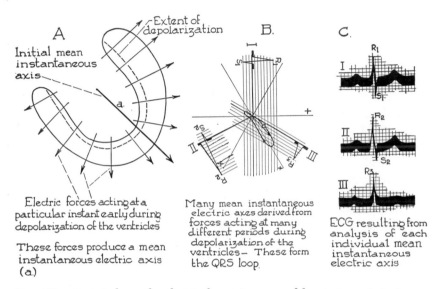

FIG. 251.—Part *A* shows the electric forces in a normal heart at one instant represented as vectors projected upon the frontal plane of the body. The septum is not shown, since under most circumstances it may be disregarded for practical purposes. (See text and Chapter 1 for details.) Part *B* shows the mean instantaneous electric axes gathered together to form the QRS loop. These forces are produced at various periods of time during inscription of the QRS complex of the electrocardiogram. (See monocardiogram or vectorcardiogram, Chapter 1, p. 62 and hapter 5, p. 249.) Part *C* shows the normal electrocardiogram.*

*In all figures to follow showing myocardial infarction, the general methods used to analyze the initial portion of the QRS complexes of the standard leads are:

1. The electric forces acting early during the depolarization of the ventricles responsible for the initial portion of the QRS complex are shown in Part *A* of Figure 252. These forces are altered by the position of the infarct.

2. The mean of these forces acting at this moment (early) is drawn and is called the *initial* mean instantaneous electric axis (Fig. 252*A*). Many such axes are inscribed during the depolarization of the ventricles. These are collected to form the QRS loop (Fig. 252*B*).

3. As the *initial* deflections of the QRS complex are important in determining the type of infarct present, only the initial portion of the complex is analyzed in detail. For simplicity, only one early mean instantaneous electric axis labeled (*a*) in the drawings is analyzed (Fig. 252*B*). In the *C* part of the figure is shown a typical electrocardiogram of the particular infarct discussed (Fig. 252*C*). The first or initial portion of the QRS complex seen in such an infarct is considered.

In the normal heart, the mean electric axis of the QRS complex is directed in the sixth sextant at an angle of about 58 degrees (Fig. 251). By analysis of the electric forces from each ventricle, which constitute the *initial mean instantaneous* electric axis, and in turn the other electric axes which make up the QRS loop, the initial portion of the QRS of the electrocardiogram can be predicted. Similarly, of course, the loop can be drawn from the QRS complexes of the electrocardiogram (Fig. 251).

In posterior myocardial infarction, the infarcted area in the posterior and diaphragmatic region leaves the electric forces acting during the

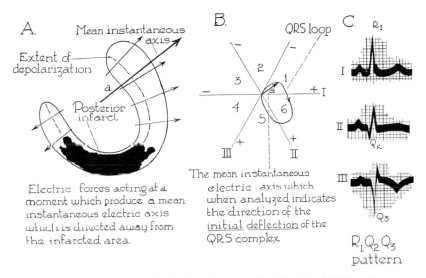

A. Mean instantaneous axis
Extent of depolarization
a
Posterior infarct

Electric forces acting at a moment which produce a mean instantaneous electric axis which is directed away from the infarcted area.

B. QRS loop

The mean instantaneous electric axis which when analyzed indicates the direction of the initial deflection of the QRS complex

C. R₁

$R_1 Q_2 Q_3$ pattern

Fɪɢ. 252.—*Posterior myocardial infarction.* An $R_1Q_2Q_3$ initial QRS pattern is produced. Part *B* shows how the first part of the QRS loop and the initial mean instantaneous electric axis (vector *a*) indicate that the initial QRS pattern is of the $R_1Q_2Q_3$ type. (See text for details.)

depolarization process at the anterolateral area of the left ventricle more or less unopposed (Fig. 252A). This produces a QRS loop with the initial portion rotated into the first sextant of the triaxial reference system (Fig. 252). Thus, if one analyzed the first part of the QRS loop for an initial mean instantaneous axis (Fig. 252B), the initial deflection of the QRS complex would show an $R_1Q_2Q_3$ pattern (Figs. 52 and 252).

On examination of the initial mean instantaneous vector, *a*, it can be seen that when a perpendicular is dropped from the terminus of the vector to the lead I line, it falls upon the positive side of the lead I line, indicating that the initial part of the QRS complex will be upright or positive, or an R wave in lead I (Fig. 252D). Figure 252C shows this to be true. A perpendicular dropped from the terminus of the vector to the lead II line falls slightly over to the negative side of this line, indicating that the initial portion of the QRS in lead II is down or negative, or a small Q wave (Fig. 252D). A perpendicular dropped from the terminus of vector a to the lead III line falls a relatively great distance to the negative side of this line, indicating that the initial portion of the QRS complex in lead III is down or negative, or a fairly large Q wave (Fig. 252C and D). Therefore, it is readily evident from what has been said that in posterior infarction the initial portion of the QRS complexes in the standard leads will be of an $R_1Q_2Q_3$ pattern. In the figures to follow concerning the initial QRS pattern in infarction, the initial mean instantaneous vector shown in the B part of the figures should be analyzed in this manner.

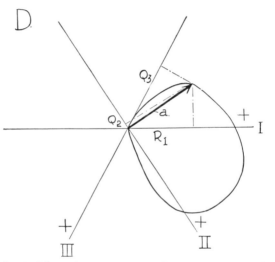

Fig. 252D.—The QRS loop shown in part B of figure 252 enlarged and analyzed to show why the initial QRS pattern is of the $R_1Q_2Q_3$ type in posterior infarction. (See text for details.)

The amplitude of the Q waves in leads II and III of the $R_1Q_2Q_3$ pattern depends upon the size of the infarct. Since the majority of posterior infarcts extend more than half way through the thickness of the wall of the ventricle, the Q_3 wave is usually greater than 0.04 second. If the Q_3 wave is half the duration of the entire QRS complex, the infarct probably extends through half the ventricular thickness. If the infarct is transmural, a single downward movement for the QRS in lead III may be inscribed. The deflection is called a QS_3 wave. Small infarcts may not exhibit electrocardiographic changes.

Anterolateral Myocardial Infarction

The main areas of the heart involved in anterolateral infarction are the anterior and lateral portions of the left ventricle. This is the region of the heart supplied by the anterior descending branch of the left coronary artery. Electrocardiographic changes in the chest leads are illustrated in figure 186. In the *limb leads* the pattern in the *initial portions* of the QRS complexes is of a $Q_1R_2R_3$ type. R_1 is often small, whereas R_2 and R_3 are frequently of large amplitude. This pattern results from the rotation of the initial segment of the QRS loop into the fourth and fifth sextants. Analysis of the electric forces of the depolarization processes in the two

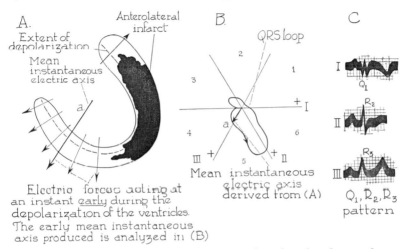

Fig. 253.—*Anterolateral myocardial infarction.* The infarct has destroyed many of the electric forces in the left ventricle. Thus, the forces in the right ventricle act almost unopposed. The initial part of the QRS loop is distorted into the fourth and fifth sextants. Analysis of the initial mean instantaneous axis (a) shows how the loop indicates the $Q_1R_2R_3$ pattern of the QRS complexes in the standard leads (part C of the figure).

ventricles and the resultant mean instantaneous electric axes in the sextants mentioned previously enable one to predict the $Q_1R_2R_3$ picture as shown in figure 253. The arguments are the same as presented for a posterior infarct.

Small Apical Myocardial Infarction
(A Type of Anterolateral Infarction)

An infarct of the anterior wall of the left ventricle, which is somewhat more apically situated than the average anterolateral infarction, throws the *initial* portion of the QRS loop into the half of the fourth sextant adjacent to the third. Thus, the initial QRS pattern is a $Q_1Q_2R_3$ pattern (Fig. 254).

Basal Myocardial Infarction
(A Type of Anterolateral Infarction)

If the infarct is located near the base of the lateral wall of the left ventricle, the *initial* QRS deflections produce a Q_1 *of low amplitude*, as the *initial* portion of the QRS loop is directed slightly into the region of the fifth sextant adjacent to the fourth (Fig. 255). The initial QRS pattern is $Q_1R_2R_3$.

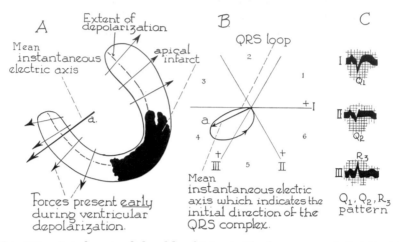

Fig. 254.—*Apical myocardial and basal infarct.* The forces are such that the initial portion of the QRS complexes present a $Q_1Q_2R_3$ pattern. (See text for explanation.) Basal component is not shown in diagram.

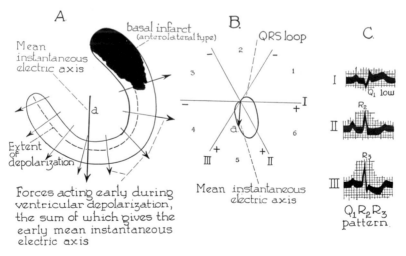

Fig. 255.—*Basal infarction.* The forces acting are mainly in the region of the apex, since the infarct has eliminated many strong forces acting in the base of the left ventricle. A low Q_1 is produced.

Strictly Anterior Myocardial Infarction

In strictly anterior infarction, the anterior portion of the septum and the adjacent portions of the anterior region of the left ventricle are the areas involved. This portion is supplied by the anterior descending branch of the left coronary artery. As the forces are acting perpendicularly to the frontal plane of the body, the standard leads are not altered and appear normal (Fig. 256). Diagnostic changes produced in the precordial leads are illustrated in figure 189.

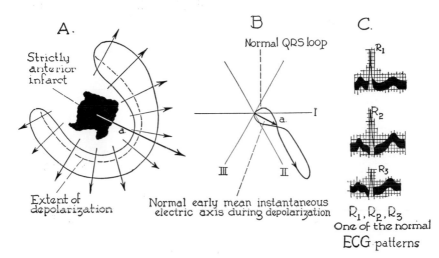

FIG. 256.—*Strictly anterior infarction.* The standard leads present no evidence of the anterior infarct.

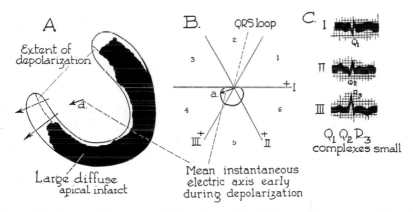

FIG. 257.—*Large, diffuse apical infarction.* The QRS complexes are small in the standard leads.

Strictly Posterior Myocardial Infarction

In a similar manner as that described for strictly anterior infarction, the standard leads reveal no evidence of a strictly posterior infarct. Changes in the precordial leads are described in figure 188.

Large, Diffuse Apical Myocardial Infarction

If the entire apex of the heart is infarcted, most of the forces in this area are destroyed, and small complexes are produced in the standard leads (Fig. 257). Precordial leads would be of diagnostic value. (See Chapter 3.) The initial pattern of the QRS is a $Q_1Q_2R_3$ type. The magnitude of the components of the QRS complex is small when compared with the small apical infarct.

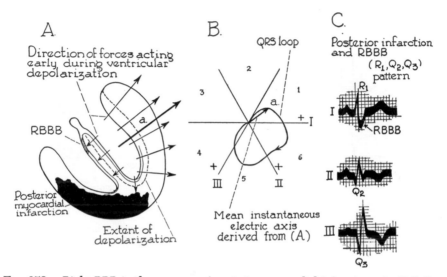

A.
Direction of forces acting early during ventricular depolarization

RBBB

Posterior myocardial infarction

Extent of depolarization

B.
QRS loop

Mean instantaneous electric axis derived from (A)

C.
Posterior infarction and RBBB
(R_1, Q_2, Q_3) pattern

I   RBBB

II Q_2

III Q_3

FIG. 258.—*Right BBB in the presence of posterior myocardial infarction. An $R_1Q_2Q_3$ initial QRS pattern results.*

MYOCARDIAL INFARCTION IN THE PRESENCE OF RIGHT BUNDLE BRANCH BLOCK

Infarction can be diagnosed in the presence of right BBB. When the right main bundle branch is blocked, the left ventricle undergoes depolarization first in essentially normal fashion. The left ventricle and septum are responsible for the recording of the initial portions of the QRS complex. Thus, myocardial infarction would have the same effect on the inscription of the initial portion of the QRS complex as if the block were not present (Fig. 258).

MYOCARDIAL INFARCTION IN THE PRESENCE OF LEFT BUNDLE BRANCH BLOCK

Myocardial infarction cannot ordinarily be diagnosed in the presence of left BBB. The initial deflections of the QRS complexes are of no diagnostic assistance, since they are distorted by the presence of the left BBB

The main initial electric forces travel, because of the blocked left bundle, in an abnormal direction and fail to allow the forces altered by the infarct to manifest themselves in a recognizable fashion in the completed electrocardiogram. Only the right ventricle is depolarized in a normal fashion in left BBB. It is the left ventricle, however, which is mainly involved with the disturbed QRS electric forces in infarction. The initial deflections of the QRS in left BBB are usually of the $R_1R_2R_3$ type. There are no Q waves. It is conceivable, however, that a $Q_1R_2R_3$ picture might be produced by the combination of left BBB and a transmural infarct of the interventricular septum.

From the foregoing discussions, it is obvious that the *QRS configurations play an important rôle in the electrocardiographic diagnosis of infarction. S–T segment and T wave changes without the characteristic QRS changes are insufficient for a definite electrocardiographic diagnosis of infarction.*

PERICARDITIS

Pericarditis has already been discussed on pages 131 and 186. It was stated that the direction of the S–T shift was indicated by a vector drawn from the centroid of the ventricle to the centroid of the injured area. Since

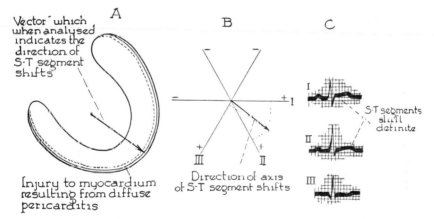

Fig. 259.—*Diffuse pericarditis.* The S–T segments are shifted up in leads I and II and are isoelectric in III. The analysis of the S–T segment "vector" is the same as for the initial electric axes in infarction previously described. There are no characteristic QRS changes in pericarditis.

pericarditis is usually found over the entire surface of the heart, the segment shifts are usually positive in leads I and II and isoelectric in III. In figure 259 it can be seen that if the arrow shown in *A* is transferred to the triaxial reference system, treated as a vector and analyzed as described previously for the mean instantaneous electric axes of the QRS in infarc-

tion, the S–T shifts in pericarditis can be predicted for the three standard leads (Fig. 259B and C).

If the pericarditis were located in an isolated area on the ventricles,
such as at the apex only, the shift would be upright, but slight, in leads
I and II and isoelectric in III (Fig. 260).

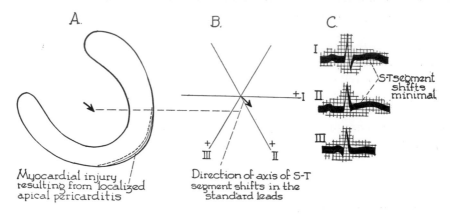

A.

B.

C.

S-Tsegment
shifts
minimal

Myocardial injury
resulting from localized
apical pericarditis

Direction of axis of S-T
segment shifts in the
standard leads

Fig. 260.—*Isolated apical pericarditis* produces the same S–T segment shifts as diffuse
pericarditis but to a smaller degree.

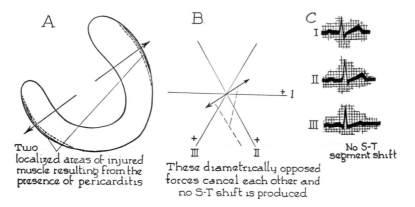

A

B.

C

No S-T
segment shift

Two
localized areas of injured
muscle resulting from the
presence of pericarditis

These diametrically opposed
forces cancel each other and
no S-T shift is produced

Fig. 261.—*Two localized areas of pericarditis,* if diametrically opposite, produce no
S–T segment shifts.

If two localized areas of pericarditis occurred which were diametrically
opposed, there would be no S–T segment shifts, because the forces produced by the currents of injury would cancel each other (Fig. 261).

Since only a superficial layer of muscle may be destroyed in pericarditis, there are no detectable changes in the electric forces during depolarization, and consequently none of the changes in the configurations of
the initial portions of the QRS complexes described for infarction are seen.

There are no QRS changes characteristic of pericarditis. This is important in the differential electrocardiographic diagnosis of acute pericarditis and myocardial infarction. The underlying myocardial ischemia produces T wave changes, however.

SPATIAL VECTORCARDIOGRAPHY

The spatial vectorcardiogram may be defined as a record of the time course in space of the mean instantaneous vectors which represent the electric activity of the heart.

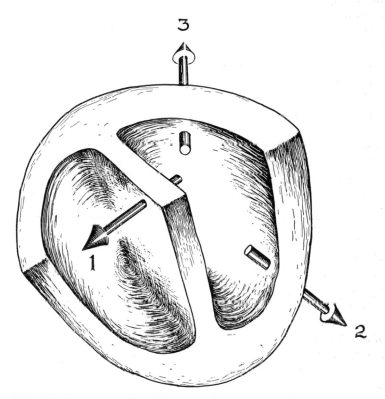

Fig. 262.—The heart is a three-dimensional structure enclosed in a volume or three-dimensional conductor, the body. Electric forces generated by the heart are oriented in space. This diagram illustrates three mean instantaneous electric vectors (1 early, 2 intermediate, and 3 late in time) from the ventricles which develop at three different moments in the cardiac cycle and are represented as vector quantities projected in space.

As indicated in Chapter 1, when the heart is depolarized and repolarized, electric currents are produced which flow in all directions in the body, a volume conductor. For example, as illustrated in figure 262, the ventricles are depolarized at various areas simultaneously, and from instant to instant the number of these areas and the configuration of the excitation wave fronts vary. The electric activity in each area individually gives rise to electric currents in the body and to potential differences within and on the surface of the body. The net currents and potential differences constitute a vector summation of the effects of the electric activity of the individual areas. For convenience in visualizing the phenomena, the electric activity in an area at any instant may be represented by an electric dipole which has direction and intensity vector characteristics. The instantaneous potential differences between points remote from the dipoles may, in turn, be considered as the effect of a resultant dipole whose direction and intensity are determined by vector addition of the individual dipole vectors. The resultant dipole is visualized as a *mean instantaneous electric vector,* which changes from instant to instant during the cardiac cycle. From measurements of the instantaneous potential differences between electrodes on the surface of the body, it is possible to determine the spatial direction and manifest magnitude of the mean instantaneous electric vector that gives rise to these potential differences. Because the heart is a volume structure and the body a volume conductor, these mean instantaneous electric vectors are directed in space, *i.e.,* they have three-dimensional orientation (Figs. 263, 264).

The magnitude and spatial direction of these mean instantaneous vectors are determined by the order of depolarization and repolarization of the auricles and ventricles and by the state of the myocardium. Because variations in the state of the myocardium with disease will alter the order of depolarization and repolarization and the magnitude and orientation of these vectors, a study of their time course (the spatial vectorcardiogram) may reveal information of clinical importance. Although such a study has not yet provided information of clinical value that cannot be obtained from the conventional electrocardiogram, there is promise that valuable data will eventually become available.

Since the original experiments of Mann, many attempts have been made recently to record accurately these mean instantaneous spatial vectors. It is almost impossible to construct them manually from the electrocardiogram with accuracy. The most satisfactory apparatus for automatically recording them is the cathode ray oscilloscope driven by suitable amplifying circuits. In addition to a suitable recorder, the location of the electrodes on the body for the recordings is extremely important in determining in part the "trueness" of the completed record. The electrodes must be placed in such positions as to permit satisfactory and easy recording of all vectors, regardless of their spatial orientation in the body.

The body and the heart possess certain intrinsic characteristics which cannot be circumvented for practical purposes. These increase the difficulties of recording, make absolutely accurate recording of the vectors impossible, and any system of electrode placement imperfect:

1. The body is not a homogeneous conductor.
2. Although the body is a volume conductor, it is irregular and finite and surrounded by air, a poor conductor.
3. Because the body is finite, the electrodes cannot be remotely placed from the source of current.
4. The heart is not a point source of current.
5. The source of current, the heart, is eccentric, and its degree of eccentricity varies during the cardiac cycle.

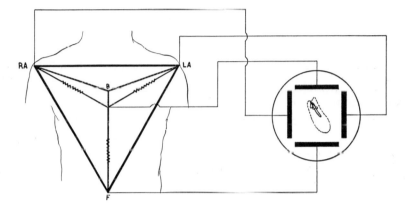

Fig. 263.—Diagrammatic representation of the equilateral tetrahedral reference system, the electrode placements on the body and the connections to the deflecting plates of the cathode ray oscilloscope for recording the *frontal plane projection* of the spatial vectorcardiogram. The standardizing factor for the horizontal deflection, right arm to left arm, is 1, whereas that for the vertical deflection, central terminal to foot, is $\sqrt{3}$ or 1.73. The connections are made in such a manner that whenever the left arm is relatively positive with respect to the right arm, the cathode ray beam is deflected toward the subject's left (viewer's right when viewing the cathode ray screen), and when the left foot is relatively positive with respect to the central terminal, the deflection is downward.

In spite of these established shortcomings, it is possible to record from points on the surface of the body the effects of the mean instantaneous electric vectors with sufficient accuracy to learn much of theoretic and possibly of clinical importance. The positions of the electrodes upon the body define a three-dimensional reference frame. Of the several reference frames suggested the *equilateral tetrahedron* of Wilson (Figs. 263 and 264) is the most accurate and certainly the most practical system available today. It has four planar surfaces, each of which forms an equilateral triangle (Figs. 263 and 264). To utilize this spatial reference system, one need only place an electrode on the back of the subject 2 cm. to the left of the spinous process of the seventh dorsal vertebra, in addition to the three electrode placements already employed in routine recording of the three standard leads (Fig. 265).

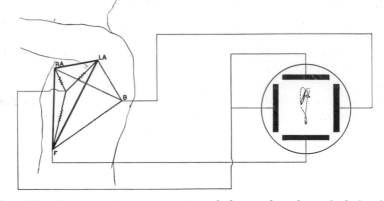

FIG. 264.—Diagrammatic representation of the equilateral tetrahedral reference system, the electrode placements on the body, and the connections to the deflecting plates of the cathode ray oscilloscope for recording the *left sagittal projection* of the spatial vectorcardiogram. The standardizing factor for the horizontal deflection, central terminal to back, is $\sqrt{3/2}$ or 1.2, whereas that for the vertical deflection, central terminal to foot, is $\sqrt{3}$ or 1.73. The connections are made in such a manner that whenever the back is relatively positive, the cathode ray beam is deflected toward the subject's back (viewer's right when viewing the cathode ray screen), and when the left foot is relatively positive with respect to the central terminal, the beam is deflected downward.

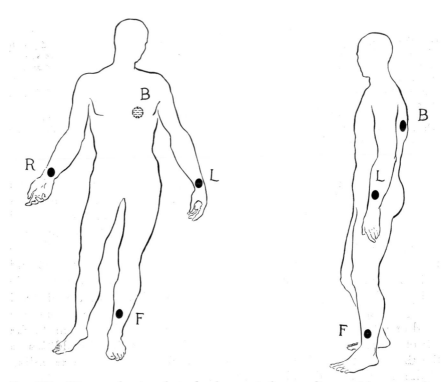

FIG. 265.—Diagram showing electrode placements for recording spatial vectorcardiogram with the equilateral tetrahedral reference system.

The equilateral tetrahedron offers the following advantages:

1. The electrodes are simple to apply and the positions are reproducible for serial recordings.
2. Only one electrode position (back) need be added to those already employed for recording the three standard leads.
3. Each of the four planar surfaces defines an *equilateral triangle*, making it possible to exploit the previous extensive work in electrocardiography based upon the equilateral triangle of Einthoven and readily permitting integration of vectorcardiography with electrocardiography.
4. The electrodes of the reference frame are adequately remote and, with use of proper standardizing factors, permit sufficiently accurate recording of the manifested spatial mean instantaneous vectors throughout the cardiac cycle to produce the spatial vectorcardiogram.

The *spatial vectorcardiogram* can be recorded stereoscopically. Details concerning circuits, timing, standardizing factors and other details necessary to obtain such recordings will not be presented here. The reference frame and standardizing factors employed during the recordings, however, must be considered when vectorcardiograms are under study.

Because the completed records are essentially closed irregular loops, the respective components have been labeled P sÊ-loop, QRS sÊ-loop, T sÊ-loop, and U sÊ-loop. The "s" connotes spatial, "Ê" an electric vector, and "P", "QRS", "T" and "U" the electric activity associated with the respective waves of the electrocardiogram.

The reader is referred to the literature for detailed information concerning spatial vectorcardiograms for normal and diseased cardiac states. Only a few selected examples of stereoscopic recordings as viewed from the frontal plane are illustrated here for orientation purposes.

The spatial vectorcardiograms of several hundred normal medical students were found, in studies employing the equilateral tetrahedral reference frame, to be of two types: Type 1 (about 80 per cent) (Fig. 266) and Type 2 (about 20 per cent) (Fig. 267). A transitional type between these two probably exists. *The wide variations in the planar projections of the spatial vectorcardiogram are the result of variations in spatial orientation of these two fundamental types.* On the basis of this observation, the stereovectorcardiogram may be used to simplify differentiation of normal and abnormal recordings.

Spatial vectorcardiography may supplement but cannot replace electrocardiography in the near future, primarily because the vectorcardiogram fails to present adequately temporal phenomena, such as cardiac rate, disturbance in rhythm, intervals between and durations of the cardiac electric activity, such as P–R and Q–T intervals, QRS duration, and so forth. Furthermore, the electrocardiogram presents similar infor-

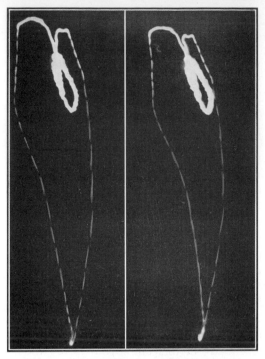

FIG. 266.—A typical Type 1 normal spatial vectorcardiogram, as viewed stereoscopically from the frontal plane. With practice, it is possible to obtain a three-dimensional image of this vectorcardiogram by holding it at a proper distance from the eyes. All spatial vectorcardiograms illustrated in this monograph were recorded with the use of the equilateral tetrahedral reference system as outlined in the text. The direction of rotation of the loops of this and all similar illustrations in this book is toward the blunt end of the dashes. There are 600 interruptions per minute.

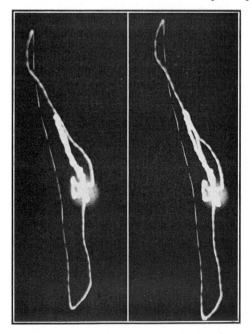

FIG. 267.—A typical Type 2 normal spatial vectorcardiogram, as viewed stereoscopically from the frontal plane. With practice, the two images can be made to fuse stereoscopically.

mation as the vectorcardiogram but in a different form. Surely, spatial vectorcardiography is worthy of study but primarily from the experimental point of view at this time. However, since the vectorcardiogram presents a detailed recording of the manifest vectors associated with the electric activity of the heart, it does provide information which is not readily, if at all, obtainable from routinely recorded electrocardiograms. For this reason, potential important information may become available from spatial vectorcardiography.

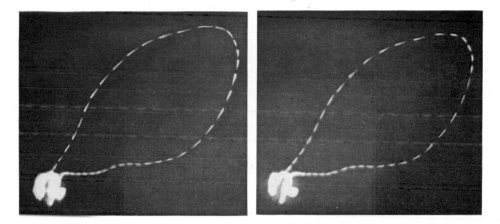

Fig. 268.—A typical spatial vectorcardiogram of left ventricular hypertrophy with myocardial ischemia, as viewed stereoscopically from the frontal plane.

The spatial vectorcardiogram observed in *left ventricular hypertrophy* with myocardial ischemia is fairly characteristic (Fig. 268). The QRS sÊ-loop is generally smooth in contour, being displaced to the subject's left shoulder and posteriorly. Its frontal plane projection is rotated counterclockwise. The T sÊ-loop is horseshoe-shaped and displaced to the subject's right, inferiorly, and anteriorly, *i.e.*, in the direction of the subject's right toes. Complicating disease states modify the general pattern. In *right ventricular hypertrophy*, the QRS sÊ-loop is displaced to the right and anteriorly to the isopotential point (Fig. 269).

The terminal portion of the QRS sÊ-loop tends to have this same displacement, and the trace tends to move slowly in *right bundle branch block* (Fig. 270). With *left bundle branch block*, the QRS sÊ-loop is displaced to the left of the isopotential point and is traced slowly, the contour of the loop tending to be irregular (Fig. 271).

An example of anterolateral infarction is illustrated in figure 272, and posterior or diaphragmatic infarction in figure 273. The vectorcardio-

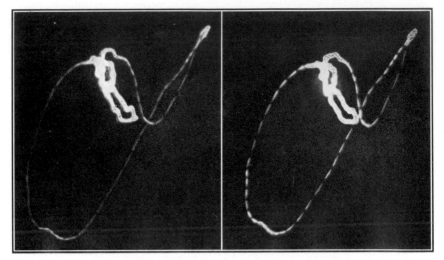

Fig. 269.—A typical spatial vectorcardiogram of right ventricular hypertrophy, as viewed stereoscopically from the frontal plane.

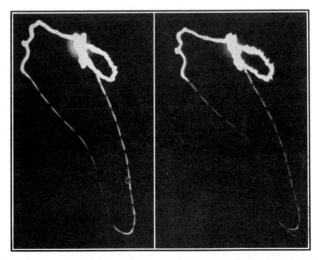

Fig. 270.—A typical spatial vectorcardiogram of right bundle branch block, as viewed stereoscopically from the frontal plane.

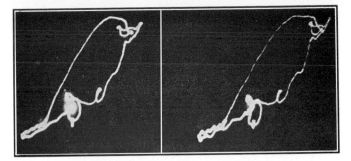

FIG. 271.—A typical spatial vectorcardiogram of left bundle branch block, as viewed stereoscopically from the frontal plane.

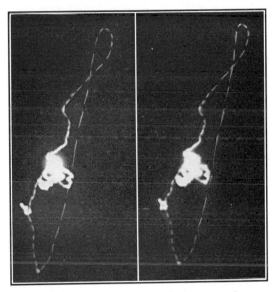

FIG. 272.—A typical spatial vectorcardiogram of anteroseptal myocardial infarction as viewed stereoscopically from the frontal plane.

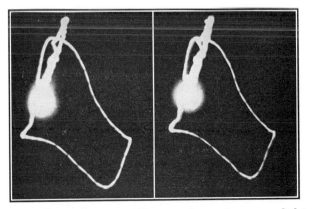

FIG. 273.—A typical spatial vectorcardiogram of posterior myocardial infarction, or infarction of the diaphragmatic wall as viewed stereoscopically from the frontal plane. The direction of rotation of the QRS sÊ-loop is clockwise.

17

gram in myocardial infarction has been discussed briefly in Chapter 5 (page 239).

The vectorcardiogram has not been accepted for general clinical application. Until a reference frame is accepted for the entire world and until the method used is simple, reliable and reproducible as well as the equipment easy to maintain, vectorcardiography will be employed only in the special centers of cardiology. Vectorcardiography also must be shown to add significantly to clinical electrocardiography with relatively little additional cost in time and effort before it can be recommended for use generally.

THE VENTRICULAR GRADIENT

The ventricular gradient was neglected for several years even though Wilson, MacLeod, Barker and Johnston (1934) had indicated the importance of the index. Ashman and his associates and Bayley have recently revived the problem by presenting more practical methods for its analysis and interpretation. Because of the importance of this parameter in clinical electrocardiography and recent interest in the subject, it is considered advisable to discuss the subject briefly by presenting the concept of the ventricular gradient without entering into any detailed discussions of its clinical applications.

It is well to consult Chapter 1 again in order to become acquainted with the concepts of depolarization and repolarization.

Definition

Differences in the time courses of depolarization and of repolarization influence the configuration of the electrocardiogram. *The net electric effect of the differences in the time courses of the processes of depolarization and repolarization* is the ventricular gradient. As defined by Wilson, the ventricular gradient indicates, in a single vector, the *net electric effect due to mean differences in the duration of the excited state.* This vector, like all vectors in electrocardiography, has *direction* in space, *magnitude,* and *sense.* Its sense is indicated by its being directed from the area in the heart in which the mean duration of the excited state is greatest to the area where the mean duration is least.

The Concept

When a hypothetical cell suspended in a volume conductor is stimulated on the right (Fig. 274), a wave of depolarization spreads over its three-dimensional surface from right to left. Figure 274 shows a depolarization wave, R wave, recorded by two galvanometers simultaneously for lead I and lead III (consult Chapter 1). If the entire system is physically and chemically homogeneous and if repolarization begins at the same point where depolarization began and spreads at a uniform rate from right to left, a wave of repolarization, T wave, will be recorded. The form and area enclosed by the T wave in each lead are the same as for the R wave in the respective lead, differing only in that its sign will be opposite. Thus, every point on the surface of the hypothetical cell remains in the excited state for precisely the same duration, and the net electric effect is zero. The algebraic sum of the R and T waves in the respective leads I and III is, therefore, zero (Fig. 274). Because there was no variation in the time courses of depolarization and repolarization or in the duration of the excited state, there was no resultant electric quantity or there was *no gradient* present.

On the other hand, the process of repolarization in the actual living cell is usually not uniform, tending to begin from several areas at one time and being relatively slow in its rate of spread. In a uniform system, repolarization generally begins where depolarization began and, therefore, spreads from right to left (Fig. 275). This results in a T wave of lower

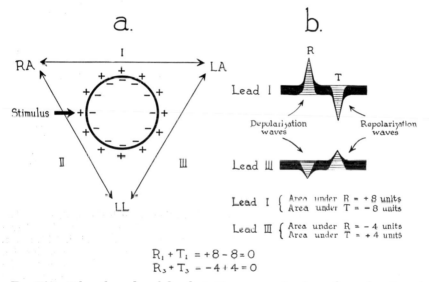

Fig. 274.—When the order of depolarization or accession is regular and uniform in rate and all portions of the "cell" remain in the excited state for an equal length of time, the order of repolarization or regression must follow the path of accession and will be regular and uniform, and the ventricular gradient will not exist.

voltage and longer duration. It encloses an area of equal magnitude but opposite in sign to the R wave. Under these circumstances, all parts of the cell did not remain in the excited state for the same length of time, even though the net electric effect due to differences in the time courses of depolarization and repolarization is zero, *i.e.*, the algebraic sum of the R and T waves is zero (Fig. 275). Thus, whereas a ventricular gradient did exist for localized areas, the over-all average electric effect was zero net, that is, the ventricular gradient existed but had a zero value.

The depolarization wave is designated the R wave and the repolarization wave the T wave, in order to draw an analogy between the hypothetic spherical cell of muscle and the human heart and between the waves of depolarization and repolarization in the hypothetic cell and those in the human electrocardiogram.

Thus, when the living cell is in the depolarized state, it is said to be in the *excited* state; when in the polarized state, it is said to be in the *resting* state. If, following the application of a stimulus, every *portion* of the cell remains in the excited state for an equal length of time, the area under the R wave must equal that under the T wave and the order of *repolarization* must retrace *exactly* the order of *depolarization*. This indicates that the

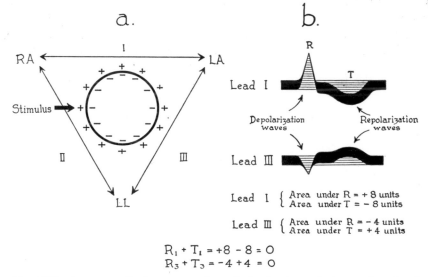

$$R_1 + T_1 = +8 - 8 = 0$$
$$R_3 + T_3 = -4 + 4 = 0$$

Fɪɢ. 275.—In most cells the process of repolarization is much slower than depolarization and tends to be irregular in order and migration. The process tends to begin where depolarization began and to terminate where depolarization ended. This results in a repolarization wave, T wave, which is of less magnitude and greater duration than the depolarization wave, R wave, certain portions of the cell remaining in the excited state longer than others. It is possible, as in this illustration, for the net electric effect due to variations in the time course of depolarization and repolarization to be zero. As a result, the area enclosed by the depolarization wave equals the area enclosed by the repolarization wave. A ventricular gradient does exist but is equal to zero.

areas under R and T must be *opposite* in sign as well as equal in magnitude. Therefore, if the values of the areas under R and T are added algebraically, the result is zero, *i.e.,* the duration of the *excited state is equal* throughout the cell. Wilson and his associates made use of this addition in order to express the *duration of the excited state* of the ventricular musculature in absolute units, which they called the *ventricular* gradient. In summary, then, the *ventricular gradient is an expression of the variations in the duration of the excited state.* Later, it will be seen that it can be represented as a vector force possessing all the mathematical characteristics of such a force.

It has been indicated in the preceding discussion that when the duration of the excited state is equal throughout in the hypothetic cell, the ventricular gradient is zero (Fig. 274), or there is *no gradient.* By neces-

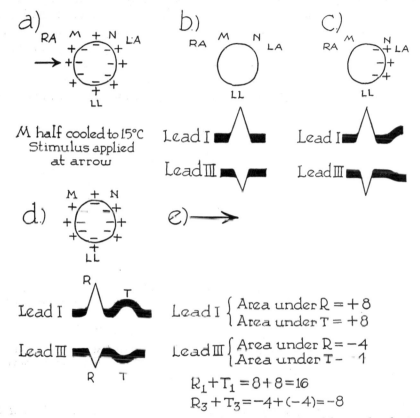

Fig. 276.—The M half of the cell was cooled to 15° C., thus delaying the physicochemical processes in the M half of the cell. When a stimulus is applied to the M half at the point indicated by the arrow, depolarization occurs relatively slowly. When the impulse reaches the N half of the cell, the depolarization process speeds up and progresses in a normal fashion (part *b* shows the cell depolarized). Since the M half is cooled, the physicochemical processes associated with recuperation and repolarization or regression are slowed so that repolarization begins on the N half of the cell (*c* part of figure), resulting in an order of regression that is opposite in direction to the order of depolarization or accession. This also produces a pronounced variation in the duration of the excited state for various portions of the cell. In this example the M half remained in the excited state for a much longer period of time than the N half. This also resulted in regression waves (T waves) with areas of the same sign as the areas of the accession waves (R waves). There is a definite *gradient.* A vector representing the gradient is directed from the point at which the mean duration of the excited state is longest to the point where it is shortest. In this example, then, it would point from the center of the M half of the cell horizontally across the center of the N half (heavy arrow *e*).

sity, the order of repolarization has retraced *exactly* the order of depolarization. Should the duration of the excited state not be uniform throughout, the ventricular gradient will have an *absolute* value and the direction and magnitude of the vector representing the gradient will be determined by the nature of these variations. For example, in figure 276, the M half of the cell has been cooled to 15° C.; this delays depolarization and particularly the rate of the reactions of the physicochemical processes leading to repolarization, so that repolarization begins on the N half first. The duration of the excited state, therefore, is not equal throughout the cell but is longer in the M half. In the resulting tracing the repolarization wave will be in the same direction as the depolarization wave and the gradient will be greater than zero, *i.e.*, it possesses an absolute value. The *vector* representing the *gradient is directed from the point in the cell in*

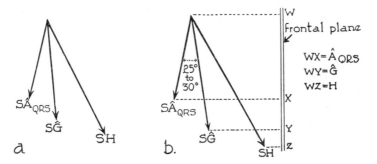

Fig. 277—(*a*) The vector forces in space of the QRS (ÂQRS) and Gradient (Ĝ) and the longitudinal anatomic axis of the heart (H) in space. (*b*) In the analysis of the standard or limb leads of the electrocardiogram only that portion of the spatial forces projected upon the frontal plane of the body are recorded. These values are called *manifest* values. For example, WX, simply called ÂQRS, is the *manifest vector* force of the spatial vector SÂQRS; WY, simply called Ĝ, is the manifest vector force of the spatial vector SĜ; and WZ, simply called H, is the manifest longitudinal anatomic axis of the spatial axis SH.

which the duration of the excited state is longest to that in which it is shortest, in this case from the right of the cell to the left, as indicated by the heavy arrow, *e* in figure 276. Obviously, if the N half of the hypothetic cell were cooled, the arrow would point from the left of the cell to the right, or if the positions of the electrodes, RA and LA, were exchanged, it would point from the left of the cell to the right. The influence of rotation of the cell will likewise affect the direction. For example, if in figure 276 the cell had been rotated clockwise through an angle of 180 degrees, the vector representing the gradient would have pointed from left to right instead of from the right of the cell to the left. Therefore, rotation of the cell, or the relationship of electrodes to each other and to the cell, will influence the direction and, obviously, the manifest magnitude (defined later) of the gradient. Again, the vector forces expressing depolarization (R wave) and repolarization (T wave) may be correlated independently with the gradient as well as with each other.

The same reasoning has been applied to the human heart. By determination of the area under the depolarization complex (QRS) and repolarization complex (T) of the human electrocardiogram and addition of these areas algebraically, the *ventricular gradient* is obtained. It has the same significance as for the hypothetic cell. *It is a vector expression (in quantitative terms) of the relative variations in duration of the excited state in the different portions of the ventricular musculature.* It is an expression of the relationship of the orders of depolarization and repolarization. *The vector representing the gradient points from the area in the heart in which the average duration of the excited state is longest to that in which it is shortest.* In the normal human heart, the direction is from endocardial to epicardial surface, and the angle it forms with the horizontal or lead I line is normally close to that of the mean electric axis of the QRS complex and close to the longitudinal anatomic axis of the heart.

Since the body and heart are volume conductors, the processes of depolarization and repolarization are directed in space and, of course, the ventricular gradient is also oriented in space. In the past, most applications of the gradient and other electric forces associated with the heart beat have been limited to projections of the spatial forces upon the frontal plane of the Einthoven triangle, but the spatial forces themselves, as well as several projected components, should be studied.

Nomenclature

From the preceding discussion it is obvious that not only is the ventricular gradient a vector force but so is the electric axis of the P, QRS, and T waves. Since the anatomic axis, the longitudinal axis of the heart drawn from the base to the apex, possesses only the quality of duration, it is obviously not a vector force. Bayley has suggested nomenclature and symbols to represent these forces in order to simplify discussions (Fig. 277). The symbols and their connotations are as follows:

G = Ventricular gradient as projected on the frontal plane of the body.

$\hat{A}_{QRS}$ = Mean manifest magnitude of the QRS complex determined algebraically and measured in microvolt seconds or units, *i.e.*, the mean force of the depolarization process of the ventricular musculature.

H = Anatomic (longitudinal) axis of the heart as projected on the frontal plane. This value has no magnitude and cannot be expressed quantitatively.

$\hat{A}_T$ = Mean manifest magnitude of the repolarization process in microvolt seconds or units.

When the arrow tip or caret (∧) is placed over the symbols, as in ÂQRS, Ĝ or ÂT, it indicates that the particular value is to be considered as a vector, *i.e.*, it has direction, magnitude, and sense. The direction is expressed in degrees accordng to the old concepts of Einthoven, *i.e.*, as the angle in degrees which the vector forms with the zero or horizontal or lead I line (Fig. 277*a*). Bayley suggested the use of the polar coordinate system of measurement, a more correct form mathematically, but because of general practice and until a new method is generally agreed upon, it is probably better to adhere to the old empiric method of expressing the direction of the vector forces in order to avoid confusion.

It is known that when the three standard leads are used, the electric forces of the heart projected on the frontal plane of the body (the manifest forces) are the ones recorded. Actually, however, these forces are extended into space away from the frontal plane. For example, the H axis projects anteriorly down and to the left; the Ĝ also points down, to the left and only slightly anteriorly, whereas the ÂQRS points down, to the left and slightly posteriorly (Fig. 277*b*). In order to represent the spatial vector, Bayley suggested that the prefix S be used as follows: SÂQRS, SÂT, or SĜ. For example, Ĝ would represent only that portion of the spatial ventricular gradient that is projected on the frontal plane, whereas SĜ would represent the entire ventricular gradient as a vector force extended into space, *i.e.*, the spatial gradient. From figure 277 it can be seen that SĜ has a greater magnitude than Ĝ, the latter being represented by the projected magnitude WY. Furthermore, SĜ has three directions; in the normal person it is directed (1) down, (2) to the left, and (3) anteriorly, whereas Ĝ has only two directions: (1) down, and (2) to the left, *i.e.*, it is considered only in one plane, along the frontal plane of the body. The spatial values are rarely used in clinical electrocardiography today. They are valuable in appreciation of the fundamental forces concerned; in fact, this concept is necessary for detailed understanding of the nature of the forces involved. The spatial force projected on the frontal plane is the force manifested by the completed electrocardiogram and is known as the *manifest* force.

Method of Measurement and Recording

Ashman and his associates have simplified the method of measuring the ventricular gradient to make it practical and still accurate enough for clincal applications. They suggested the following procedure. The areas of the QRS and T (the depolarization and repolarization complexes) are determined as shown graphically in figure 278. The areas above the isoelectric line are positive values and those below negative. The areas are determined by counting the "squares" formed by the millimeter and time lines or by measuring the height of a complex in microvolts and multiplying this factor by one-half the width of the base in seconds. One millimeter is equal to 100 microvolts in a properly standardized electrocardiogram. A lens for magnification aids in these measurements. The units are expressed in microvolt seconds. Each time line is 0.04 second apart and each millimeter line represents 100 microvolts with the usual standardization; therefore, each small rectangular division on the tracing represents 4 microvolt seconds (4 μv.s., often referred to as *one*

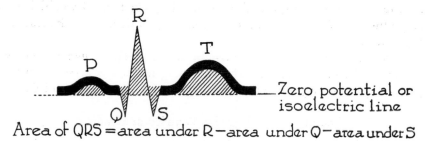

Fig. 278.—Diagram showing the areas measured to determine the area under the QRS complex and the area under the 'T' wave. Areas above the isoelectric line are considered to be positive values and those below negative.

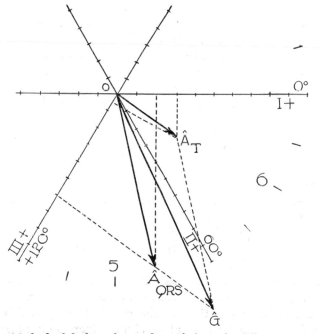

Fig. 279.—Method of finding the gradient $\hat{G}$ from the following values: QRS in lead I = +2 units, QRS in lead III = +6 units, T in lead I = +3 units, T in lead III = +0.5 unit. $\hat{G}$ has a magnitude of 12.5 units and a direction of +65°. $\hat{A}_{QRS}$ and $\hat{A}_T$ were first found as described in the text. Then $\hat{G}$ was found by means of the parallelogram law of analysis of vector forces.

unit). The algebraic addition of the positive and negative values is equal to the net area of the QRS and T or net magnitude of the depolarization and repolarization processes, respectively. A planimeter may be used for more accurate, but less practical, measurements.

In order to find Ĝ, one finds ÂQRS and ÂT from any two leads, preferably leads I and III, by obtaining the algebraic sum of the areas of QRS and T for the leads, and adds them as vector quantities. For example, suppose the net area of the QRS in lead I is +2 and in lead III +6 and the net area of T in lead I is +3 and in lead III +0.5; then G would have a magnitude of 12.5 units and a direction of +65 degrees, as indicated in figure 279.

More cumbersome methods have been employed to increase the accuracy of the measurements. The foregoing method is accurate to ±15 per cent for the magnitude and ±5 degrees for the direction of Ĝ.

Factors Influencing the Ventricular Gradient

Certain factors will influence the direction and magnitude of the ventricular gradient. These factors, some of which are included hereafter, are important in health and in disease.

Rotation of the heart about its anteroposterior axis will change the ventricular gradient. Rotation *counterclockwise* (rotation to the *left*) will rotate the axis of Ĝ to the left and make it transverse. The axis G is rotated more than the anatomic axis of the heart. A rotation to the *right*, or *clockwise* rotation, will make Ĝ vertical, *i.e.*, Ĝ will rotate to the right. The range of normal rotation of Ĝ is greater than that of the anatomic axis (H) but not as great as that of ÂQRS.

Rotation of the heart about its longitudinal axis will change the ventricular gradient. From figures 277*b* and 282, it is obvious that rotation of the heart about the H axis (longitudinal anatomic axis) will change the relationship of the axis of Ĝ, QRS, and H. In normal subjects the axis of the gradient should not be more than 24 degrees to the right of the QRS axis and not more than 35 degrees to the left of it.

The influence of *rotation of the heart about its transverse axis* upon the gradient is not well understood.

Posture, in large part, by its influence on cardiac position, will alter the gradient. Standing decreases the magnitude of the gradient and tends to rotate it to the right.

Cardiac rate will modify the magnitude and direction of the gradient (Fig. 280). An increase in rate will tend to decrease the magnitude of its manifest area. These variations in the gradient are probably related to many physiologic changes associated with the increase in pulse rate.

Normal variations in direction and magnitude of the gradient (Ĝ) are shown in figure 281. Ĝ may normally extend slightly into the first sextant.

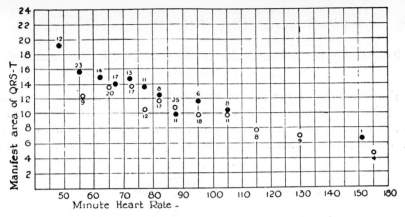

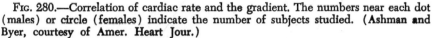

FIG. 280.—Correlation of cardiac rate and the gradient. The numbers near each dot (males) or circle (females) indicate the number of subjects studied. (Ashman and Byer, courtesy of Amer. Heart Jour.)

Deviation of A_{QRS} with respect to
the normal ventricular gradient
Max. $+\angle$ = 24°, Mag = 11·48 MVS
Max. $-\angle$ = -35°, Mag = 10·80 MVS

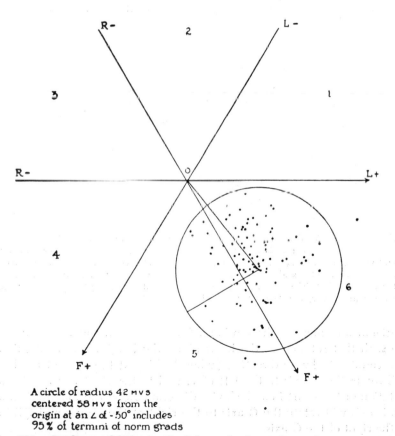

A circle of radius 42 MVS
centered 58 MVS from the
origin at an $\angle$ of -50° includes
95% of termini of norm grads

FIG. 281.—Gradients of 100 normal adults. The dots indicate the termini of the gradients. (Bayley, courtesy of Amer. Heart Jour.)

Relationship of the Ventricular Gradient to the QRS Axis and to the Longitudinal Anatomic Axis of the Heart

The directions of the axis of the gradient and QRS axis are closely related in the normal subject, as shown in figure 282. The two axes tend to follow each other rather closely and fall more or less within the range previously stated. From careful study of figure 282, it can be seen that the

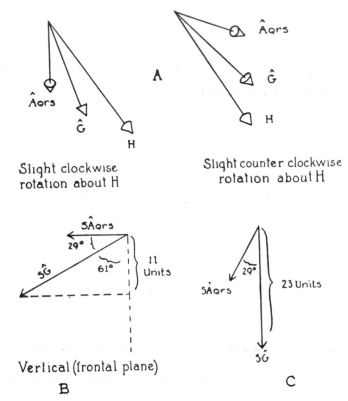

FIG. 282.—A, Correlation of the spatial and manifest axes of the ÂQRS, Ĝ, and H axes as influenced by rotation of the heart. B, The spatial axes as seen in a right lateral view when the axes lie in a sagittal plane. The vertical dotted line marks the intersection of frontal and sagittal planes. C, The spatial electric axes after rotation of the heart so that SĜ marks the intersection of frontal and sagittal planes. (Ashman, Gardberg and Byer, courtesy of Amer. Heart Jour.)

spatial arrangement of the QRS and Ĝ axes about the anatomic axis (H) are such that rotation of the heart along the longitudinal anatomic axis in a counterclockwise direction (when looking at the apex of the heart) will rotate the Ĝ axis to the left of H and to the right of the QRS axis. Rotation of the heart in a clockwise direction along the longitudinal anatomic axis will rotate the Ĝ axis to the right of the H axis and QRS axis to the right of the Ĝ axis.

Normal Values of the Gradient

The manifest magnitude of Ĝ averages 13.0 units; 1 unit is equal to 4 microvolt seconds. It is slightly greater in men than in women. The magnitude of Â$_{QRS}$ is 5.9 units in women and 6.7 units in men, *i.e.*, Ĝ is about double Â$_{QRS}$. A 50 per cent increase in cardiac rate decreases the

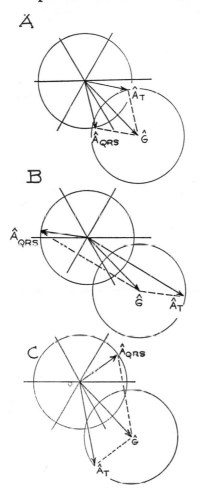

Fɪɢ. 283.—Illustration showing the rotation of Â$_{QRS}$ around the origin of the triaxial reference system. When Ĝ is fixed, there results an inscription of a similar figure by the terminus of Â$_T$ around the terminus Ĝ as a center with Â$_T$ rotated 180° away from Â$_{QRS}$. Parts A, B, and C show Â$_{QRS}$ rotated in three different positions about the center of the triaxial reference system, with Â$_T$ having necessarily rotated into three different positions respectively, in order to maintain the same Ĝ. Thus, it is seen that as the terminus of Â$_{QRS}$ describes a circle around the center of the triaxial reference system, the terminus of Â$_T$ describes a circle around the terminus Ĝ as a center. Although a circle is described in the figure for simplicity of illustration, regardless of the shape of the trace described by the terminus of Â$_{QRS}$ about the center of the triaxial system, a similar figure will be described by the terminus of Â$_T$ around the terminus of Ĝ.

magnitude of Ĝ about 39 per cent. The maximal magnitude of Ĝ is probably not known, but normally it is near 23.0 units, and the minimal is about 2.5 units. The maximal magnitude of ÂQRS is about 12.0 units and the minimal about —3.5 units.

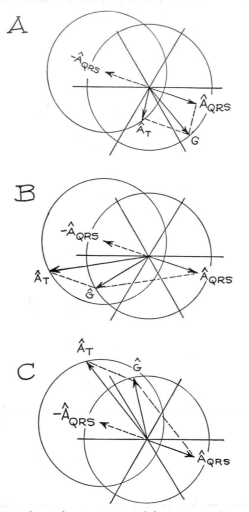

Fig. 284.—Illustration shows that as rotation of the terminus Ĝ around the center of the triaxial reference system describes a trace when ÂQRS remains fixed, the terminus of ÂT traces a similar figure around —ÂQRS with its terminus as the center. Parts A, B, and C show the Ĝ rotated into three different positions around the origin of the triaxial reference system and ÂQRS fixed in the same position. Thus, the terminus of ÂT is seen to inscribe a similar figure around the terminus of —ÂQRS as the terminus of Ĝ described around the origin of the triaxial reference system; regardless of the configuration of the trace made by the terminus of ÂQRS, the terminus of ÂT will inscribe a similar one around the terminus of —ÂQRS. From this figure and the preceding one, it is possible to distinguish secondary from primary T wave changes. When these vectors fail to fill such a relationship, then primary T wave changes exist.

Ĝ normally forms an angle of +20 degrees or less with the longitudinal anatomic axis (H). Ĝ rarely is found normally outside of 0 degree and +90 degrees, *i.e.*, it is rarely outside the sixth and adjacent half of the fifth sextants of the triaxial reference system (Fig. 285). As previously mentioned, Ĝ normally lies not over 24 degrees to the right of ÂQRS and 35 degrees to the left of ÂQRS.

If the terminus of ÂQRS describes an arbitrary path about 0, the center, in the triaxial reference system, while Ĝ remains fixed, the terminus of ÂT describes a similar path (appearing as if rotated through 180 degrees) about the terminus of Ĝ. The path of ÂT thus describes all possible variations of ÂQRS (Fig. 283). If the terminus of Ĝ is made to describe an arbitrary path about 0 while ÂQRS remains fixed, the terminus of ÂT describes a similar path about the terminus of —ÂQRS. The path of ÂT describes any variations in ÂT due to all possible variations in Ĝ (Fig. 284). These rules make it possible to distinguish primary from secondary T wave changes, an important differentiation.

The effects of drugs, fainting, and other factors have been studied but will not be discussed here.

Clinical Application of the Ventricular Gradient

In disease, the ventricular gradient is altered in magnitude and direction, as well as in its relationship to the axis of the QRS and the anatomic axis (H), for disease will disturb the orders of depolarization and repolarization and the duration of the excited state. For example, it is possible to interpret the significance of the T wave changes in the electrocardiogram with the use of the gradient. T wave changes secondary to changes in the position of the heart will possess a normal gradient in all respects, whereas if primary T wave changes occur as a result of disease of the myocardium, the gradient will be abnormal in its magnitude, direction, or relation to the other axes. At times, all three changes are present simultaneously. For example, coronary occlusion, which produces primary T wave changes, will characteristically alter the gradient. In strictly apical myocardial infarction, the gradient is shorter or even reversed and is located in the third sextant, whereas a diffuse basal infarction will produce a gradient of excessive magnitude. In general, ischemia of the heart due to impairment of the circulation through the right coronary artery will produce rotation of Ĝ to the left or within the first or second sextant, whereas ischemia of that portion of the heart supplied by the left coronary artery will rotate Ĝ to the right or into the fifth sextant.

When there is doubt about many changes in the electrocardiogram, such as low or negative T waves in lead I in clinically normal persons, the gradient is of paramount assistance in determining the clinical significance of such T waves.

If there is a greater than normal deviation in the angles between the Â$_{QRS}$ and Ĝ and H axes than would be expected on rotation of the heart alone, it is safe to conclude that there is disease of the myocardium. Such questions frequently arise in subjects with vertical or transverse hearts, in whom changes produced by rotation and disease are difficult to differentiate.

It is impossible in a monograph of this type to present detailed explanations for changes in the gradient with each type of disease. With a knowledge of the fundamental concept of the gradient, one can develop such explanations.

DIAGNOSTIC VALUE OF THE ELECTROCARDIOGRAM

At this point it is desirable to indicate the value and limitations of the electrocardiogram in the cardiac examination. A meticulously thorough history and a *careful, complete physical examination* are of the greatest value in the study of the heart. The *electrocardiogram,* the *roentgenographic* or *fluoroscopic examination,* and other laboratory data are indispensable supplementary data of much less importance.

The electrocardiographic observations *do not establish an etiologic diagnosis.* It will be recalled that there are four electrocardiographic interpretations that are usually made, none of which indicate the etiologic diagnosis (page 231, paragraph 6). It may sometimes be said that the electrocardiogram is *compatible* with mitral stenosis if there is right ventricular hypertrophy, a prolonged P–R interval, and high, wide, notched P waves, but pulmonary stenosis may also produce this same pattern. The tracing is diagnostic of neither. In the case of coronary occlusion, the electrocardiogram does not indicate the etiology of the occlusion. It may be due to syphilis, arteriosclerosis, thrombo-angiitis obliterans, or periarteritis nodosum, but the electrocardiogram may be definitely diagnostic of myocardial infarction and, as discussed previously, may sharply localize the infarct.

The electrocardiogram *does not indicate the prognosis.* The cardiac prognosis should be made by the clinician who examines both the electrocardiogram and the patient and *not by the electrocardiographer,* who examines only the tracing. If the tracing shows complete auriculoventricular block, the electrocardiographer, as well as the clinician, knows that about 75 per cent of patients with such a tracing die within a few months and that such a patient will rarely live several years. The clinician is better able to determine the prognosis than the electrocardiographer, and it is neither necessary nor expected that the electrocardiographer give a prognosis. Likewise, it is well known that in patients with coronary occlusion the electrocardiographic pattern may be reverting to normal but the patient may be dying with rapid progression of congestive heart failure.

A clinician who collects the clinical data and reads the electrocardiogram himself can treat his patient best.

The electrocardiogram *does not indicate the presence of valvular disease.* A patient with pulmonary stenosis may have an electrocardiographic pattern that is identical with that in pulmonary hypertension. Valvular lesions, like all cardiac lesions, are identified clinically after much careful study by all methods available, the electrocardiogram being one important procedure.

The electrocardiogram *does not indicate the state of compensation of the heart or the state of the cardiac reserve.* It *does not* record mechanical cardiac events, only electric events.

Remember that *a patient may have a normal electrocardiogram and still have serious cardiac disease.* He may walk out of the heart station with a normal electrocardiogram in his hand and drop dead of cardiac failure. On the other hand, *if the tracing is definitely abnormal, the patient has cardiac disease,* regardless of all other clinical data.

The electrocardiogram is especially useful in:

1. Determining the *cardiac mechanism.*

2. Indicating the presence of myocardial change, in particular, myocardial death resulting from *coronary occlusion.*

3. Indicating the presence of myocardial injury and ischemia, as in *angina pectoris.*

4. Showing the effect of drugs, such as *digitalis* and its derivatives.

5. Showing the presence of *right* or *left ventricular hypertrophy.*

6. Presenting evidence of defects in the *conduction* of impulses in the heart.

7. Indicating myocardial disease of a general nature.

8. Establishing an *etiologic, anatomic,* and *physiologic* cardiac diagnosis and prognosis when considered along with the *other clinical data.*

9. Aiding in the treatment of cardiac disease.

*   *   *   *   *

NO CARDIAC STUDY IS COMPLETE WITHOUT AN ELECTROCARDIOGRAM

APPENDIX

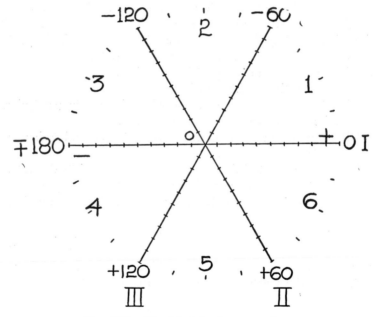

FIG. 285.—The triaxial reference system.

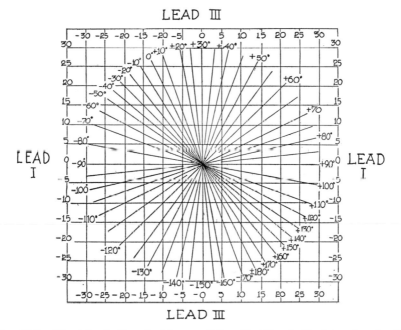

FIG. 286.—*Chart for finding electric axes* (Dieuaide Chart). *To determine the electric axis of the QRS complex:* The algebraic sum of the positive and negative deflections of the QRS complex in lead I is plotted along the lead I line (ordinate), and the algebraic sum of the positive and negative deflections of the QRS complex in lead III is plotted along the lead III line (abscissa). Perpendicular lines are drawn to these points. The point of junction of these perpendiculars represents the tip of the arrowhead of a vector force of the QRS axis, the tail being at zero or center of the graph. The angle can be determined from the angle of the axes in the graph nearest the vector formed. The same procedure is employed to find the electric axis of the *T wave* or any component of the electrocardiogram. (See Chapter 1.)

Tables 2 through 13 represent twelve "sets" of tables of normal values for amplitude, duration and ratio of amplitudes of various complexes of the electrocardiogram according to age. (From: *Electrocardiography in the Diagnosis of Congenital Heart Disease*, Burch, G. E. and DePasquale, N. P., Lea & Febiger, 1966.)

TABLE 2
AMPLITUDE (mm.)

		I	II	III	V_1	V_6
P	Mean	0.8	1.2	0.7	0.9	
	Range	0.2 / 1.6	0.4 / 2.5	0.2 / 2.2	−1.0 / 2.5	
	P_{90}	1.2	1.8	1.2	1.9	
Q	Mean	0.4		1.5		0.5
	Range	0.1 / 1.2		0.2 / 4.6		0.1 / 1.5
	P_{90}	0.7		2.7		0.9

0 — 1 Week
(126 Subjects)

AMPLITUDE (mm.)

		I	II	III	V_{3R}	V_1	V_2	V_4	V_5	V_6
R	Mean	1.5	4.0	6.0	6.8	7.6	10.2	7.5		3.0
	Range	0.2 / 3.6	0.3 / 10.0	1.5 / 13.7	1.5 / 13.0	2.5 / 17.9	3.2 / 25.0	2.0 / 14.0		0.2 / 6.5
	P_{90}	2.4	6.5	9.5	10.6	12.0	15.3	12.2		4.6
S	Mean	4.2	2.6	1.7	2.0	2.6	9.9	6.9		2.9
	Range	0.8 / 10.0	0.2 / 6.7	0.1 / 5.0	0.2 / 6.5	0.2 / 12.0	1.0 / 20.8	0.8 / 19.0		0.3 / 11.0
	P_{90}	6.8	4.6	2.8	3.7	5.2	16.6	12.1		4.5

DURATION (sec.)

	Mean	Range	S.D.
P_{II}	0.059	0.040 / 0.080	0.010
P-R Seg. Lead II	0.049	0.022 / 0.072	0.012
P-R Int. Lead II	0.108	0.078 / 0.152	0.015
QRS	0.062	0.040 / 0.082	0.009
Q-T	0.284	0.182 / 0.355	0.050
Int. Def. V_1	0.021	0.010 / 0.040	0.005
Int. Def. V_6	0.017	0.005 / 0.030	0.005

RATIO

	Mean	Range	P_{90}
R:S in V_1	7.0	1.0 / 41.5	13.0
R:S in V_6	2.3	0.1 / 11.3	

TABLE 3
AMPLITUDE (mm.)

		I	II	III	V₁	V₆
P	Mean	0.9	1.2	0.8	0.9	
	Range	0.0 1.6	0.5 2.0	-0.2 1.8	-0.5 2.6	
	P₉₀	1.4	1.8	1.4	2.1	
Q	Mean	0.5		1.2		1.5
	Range	0.1 3.2		0.1 5.0		0.1 3.6
	P₉₀	1.0		2.9		2.1

1 Week — 1 Month
(60 Subjects)

AMPLITUDE (mm.)

		I	II	III	V₃ᵣ	V₁	V₂	V₄	V₅	V₆
R	Mean	3.4	6.2	7.5	9.8	11.5	17.7	14.2	12.3	7.2
	Range	0.5 9.0	1.0 15.0	1.0 16.0	1.8 17.5	3.0 23.0	6.8 28.3	9.9 22.1	1.0 31.0	1.0 22.0
	P₉₀	5.5	11.0	11.7	15.0	17.0	25.4	19.6	20.0	11.3
S	Mean	3.2	2.8	1.4	4.1	6.2	9.1	5.9	4.2	2.2
	Range	1.0 6.3	0.2 5.5	0.1 5.0	0.2 8.2	0.3 14.5	3.6 15.3	2.0 11.4	0.5 13.0	0.1 10.0
	P₉₀	5.2	4.5	2.0	6.6	8.9	10.8	8.2	8.6	5.5

DURATION (sec.)

	Mean	Range	S.D.
Pᵢᵢ	0.048	0.320 0.080	0.018
P-R Seg. Lead II	0.048	0.022 0.074	0.014
P-R Int. Lead II	0.096	0.076 0.142	0.018
QRS	0.060	0.041 0.080	0.008
Q-T	0.240	0.186 0.300	0.048
Int. Def. V₁	0.020	0.005 0.032	0.004
Int. Def. V₆	0.022	0.010 0.033	0.005

RATIO

	Mean	Range	P₉₀
R:S in V₁	3.6	0.2 18.5	5.0
R:S in V₆	6.7	1.5 15.0	

TABLE 4
AMPLITUDE (mm.)

		I	II	III	V$_1$	V$_6$
P	Mean	0.9	1.3	0.7	1.0	
	Range	0.0 2.0	0.7 2.1	0.4 1.8	−0.2 2.5	
	P$_{90}$	1.8	1.9	1.6	2.0	
Q	Mean	0.6		1.4		1.5
	Range	0.1 2.8		0.1 5.6		0.1 3.8
	P$_{90}$	1.3		3.5		2.4

1 Month — 3 Months
(62 Subjects)

AMPLITUDE (mm.)

		I	II	III	V$_{3R}$	V$_1$	V$_2$	V$_4$	V$_5$	V$_6$
R	Mean	6.2	10.4	7.5	6.8	9.0	13.4	13.7	14.2	8.7
	Range	1.5 15.0	2.0 20.0	1.5 16.0	2.0 15.0	1.5 18.0	7.9 19.0	7.8 21.5	3.5 23.5	2.0 16.0
	P$_{90}$	10.5	15.0	11.4	12.5	14.5	17.2	16.2	17.0	10.5
S	Mean	3.6	2.9	1.6	3.8	6.1	8.3	7.9	6.6	3.2
	Range	1.6 7.4	1.7 6.0	0.2 4.2	0.2 8.5	0.1 16.0	4.3 13.2	4.6 10.8	0.5 14.5	0.1 7.0
	P$_{90}$	6.0	3.8	2.5	7.0	9.0	11.8	9.2	10.5	4.5

DURATION (sec.)

	Mean	Range	S.D.
P$_{II}$	0.051	0.036 0.086	0.016
P-R Seg. Lead II	0.050	0.024 0.076	0.012
P-R Int. Lead II	0.101	0.080 0.142	0.015
QRS	0.061	0.048 0.080	0.009
Q-T	0.248	0.180 0.346	0.045
Int. Def. V$_1$	0.021	0.010 0.032	0.005
Int. Def. V$_6$	0.024	0.015 0.034	0.006

RATIO

	Mean	Range	P$_{90}$
R:S in V$_1$	2.4	0.3 9.2	4.2
R:S in V$_6$	7.5	1.1 14.5	

TABLE 5
AMPLITUDE (mm.)

		I	II	III	V₁	V₆	
	Mean	0.9	1.3	0.8	0.7		3 Months — 6 Months
P	Range	0.2 1.7	0.9 2.2	−0.2 1.7	0.5 2.0		(66 Subjects)
	P₉₀	1.5	2.0	1.4	1.8		
	Mean	0.5		2.6		1.9	
Q	Range	0.1 2.2		0.1 6.3		0.1 4.0	
	P₉₀	1.2		3.9		2.9	

AMPLITUDE (mm.)

		I	II	III	V₃ᵣ	V₁	V₂	V₄	V₅	V₆
	Mean	7.1	11.0	7.6	6.5	8.6	14.5	15.7	15.2	9.8
R	Range	1.5 14.8	3.5 21.2	1.8 17.5	3.0 12.0	3.0 19.0	9.6 21.6	8.5 22.7	4.2 26.0	4.5 21.5
	P₉₀	10.6	14.0	13.4	9.1	15.1	18.8	18.0	19.7	15.5
	Mean	3.4	1.7	1.4	3.1	5.2	10.7	7.5	5.2	1.8
S	Range	1.1 6.0	0.2 3.9	0.1 3.2	0.8 6.0	2.0 11.2	1.5 16.0	4.5 11.0	0.5 15.2	0.1 6.2
	P₉₀	5.2	2.5	2.2	4.8	9.0	14.2	8.9	9.5	4.6

DURATION (sec.)

	Mean	Range	S.D.
Pᵢᵢ	0.058	0.040 0.082	0.022
P-R Seg. Lead II	0.046	0.026 0.080	0.010
P-R Int. Lead II	0.104	0.080 0.140	0.015
QRS	0.066	0.050 0.085	0.008
Q-T	0.248	0.200 0.360	0.042
Int. Def. V₁	0.024	0.005 0.034	0.006
Int. Def. V₆	0.029	0.020 0.040	0.007

RATIO

	Mean	Range	P₉₀
R:S in V₁	2.1	0.3 5.0	3.3
R:S in V₆	8.2	1.7 16.5	

TABLE 6
AMPLITUDE (mm.)

		I	II	III	V₁	V₆
	Mean	0.9	1.1	0.7	0.4	
P	Range	0.4 / 2.0	0.5 / 2.0	−0.4 / 1.5	0.2 / 1.8	
	P_{90}	1.6	1.9	1.2	1.3	
	Mean	0.7		2.3		2.6
Q	Range	0.1 / 3.2		0.1 / 6.0		0.2 / 5.8
	P_{90}	1.4		3.7		3.2

6 Months — 1 Year
(65 Subjects)

AMPLITUDE (mm.)

		I	II	III	V₃ᵣ	V₁	V₂	V₄	V₅	V₆
	Mean	7.4	10.8	7.2	5.0	8.5	14.5	17.2	14.8	12.7
R	Range	2.0 / 15.8	4.4 / 20.0	1.2 / 15.8	2.8 / 9.0	3.2 / 22.3	4.0 / 22.3	9.1 / 27.0	7.0 / 28.5	4.0 / 23.0
	P_{90}	11.0	14.0	12.3	8.5	12.0	17.8	25.2	19.7	16.5
	Mean	3.0	2.2	2.5	3.9	5.4	11.2	6.9	4.2	2.6
S	Range	0.2 / 8.0	0.1 / 4.6	0.1 / 8.0	1.6 / 7.0	1.5 / 17.5	3.4 / 17.6	1.0 / 10.8	0.2 / 16.0	0.7 / 8.6
	P_{90}	5.8	3.0	3.2	5.8	10.5	16.5	7.5	7.3	5.5

DURATION (sec.)

	Mean	Range	S.D.
P_{II}	0.060	0.042 / 0.086	0.018
P-R Seg. Lead II	0.050	0.030 / 0.082	0.014
P-R Int. Lead II	0.110	0.080 / 0.146	0.016
QRS	0.068	0.048 / 0.084	0.009
Q-T	0.268	0.200 / 0.320	0.044
Int. Def. V₁	0.020	0.010 / 0.032	0.005
Int. Def. V₆	0.030	0.020 / 0.044	0.008

RATIO

	Mean	Range	P_{90}
R:S in V₁	2.0	0.2 / 5.9	3.0
R:S in V₆	8.5	1.4 / 16.4	

TABLE 7
AMPLITUDE (mm.)

		I	II	III	V₁	V₆
P	Mean	1.0	1.3	0.7	0.6	
P	Range	0.4 1.5	0.6 2.3	−0.3 1.4	0.3 1.8	
P	P_{90}	1.4	2.0	1.1	1.6	
Q	Mean	0.4		2.6		1.5
Q	Range	0.1 3.0		0.2 8.8		0.1 5.4
Q	P_{90}	1.8		4.1		2.7

1 Year — 3 Years
(88 Subjects)

AMPLITUDE (mm.)

		I	II	III	V₃ᵣ	V₁	V₂	V₄	V₅	V₆
R	Mean	6.9	10.1	6.1	4.4	6.5	11.8	14.2	14.2	12.9
R	Range	1.8 16.0	5.0 19.5	0.8 13.8	1.0 9.0	2.0 17.5	4.4 20.0	4.2 26.2	6.8 30.0	5.0 25.4
R	P_{90}	10.0	14.1	11.6	7.1	11.0	16.4	19.2	19.5	19.0
S	Mean	2.1	2.0	1.9	4.7	7.4	11.8	7.0	3.8	2.8
S	Range	0.4 5.2	0.2 8.6	0.5 4.4	1.0 11.2	1.0 24.0	4.0 21.0	0.5 16.2	0.6 10.5	0.2 8.5
S	P_{90}	4.2	5.4	3.8	7.3	12.5	19.4	8.4	6.5	4.8

DURATION (sec.)

	Mean	Range	S.D.
Pᵢᵢ	0.073	0.057 0.088	0.031
P-R Seg. Lead II	0.056	0.030 0.087	0.018
P-R Int. Lead II	0.129	0.082 0.148	0.022
QRS	0.068	0.042 0.086	0.012
Q-T	0.270	0.200 0.340	0.062
Int. Def. V₁	0.019	0.010 0.040	0.006
Int. Def. V₆	0.031	0.015 0.046	0.004

RATIO

	Mean	Range	P_{90}
R:S in V₁	1.2	0.2 5.0	1.8
R:S in V₆	8.6	1.9 14.3	

Table 8
AMPLITUDE (mm.)

		I	II	III	V_1	V_6
	Mean	0.8	1.0	0.5	0.8	
P	Range	0.5 1.3	0.2 2.2	−0.2 1.1	0.1 2.2	
	P_{90}	1.1	2.0	0.9	1.6	
	Mean	0.8		2.1		1.4
Q	Range	0.1 2.2		0.1 5.5		0.1 4.8
	P_{90}	1.3		3.6		2.8

3 Years — 5 Years
(80 Subjects)

AMPLITUDE (mm.)

		I	II	III	V_{3R}	V_1	V_2	V_4	V_5	V_6
	Mean	7.6	11.7	6.4	4.0	5.9	11.1		10.0	13.1
R	Range	1.2 18.0	1.3 21.2	0.2 17.6	1.0 7.0	0.8 13.2	6.0 20.0		5.0 14.0	3.8 25.5
	P_{90}	11.3	16.3	12.5	6.2	9.5	14.2		13.5	21.1
	Mean	1.9	1.7	1.5	4.0	9.4	15.5		3.0	2.5
S	Range	0.2 5.7	0.1 4.0	0.2 6.0	1.0 8.0	2.2 21.0	5.5 27.0		0.8 9.0	0.2 9.0
	P_{90}	4.5	3.4	3.2	5.7	15.2	20.0		5.4	5.0

DURATION (sec.)

	Mean	Range	S.D.
P_{II}	0.075	0.048 0.110	0.140
P-R Seg. Lead II	0.049	0.029 0.073	0.013
P-R Int. Lead II	0.124	0.010 0.170	0.026
QRS	0.072	0.042 0.090	0.011
Q-T	0.288	0.220 0.368	0.049
Int. Def. V_1	0.018	0.010 0.030	0.006
Int. Def. V_6	0.032	0.018 0.042	0.006

RATIO

	Mean	Range	P_{90}
R:S in V_1	0.7	0.1 2.5	1.2
R:S in V_6	7.7	1.3 19.0	

TABLE 9
AMPLITUDE (mm.)

		I	II	III	V_1	V_6
P	Mean	0.8	1.2	0.6	0.9	
	Range	0.3 / 1.1	0.8 / 2.1	−0.2 / 1.3	0.2 / 2.0	
	P_{90}	1.0	1.9	1.0	1.8	
Q	Mean	0.4		1.3		1.2
	Range	0.2 / 3.0		0.2 / 3.0		0.2 / 4.5
	P_{90}	1.4		2.1		2.5

5 Years — 8 Years
(61 Subjects)

AMPLITUDE (mm.)

		I	II	III	V_{3R}	V_1	V_2	V_4	V_5	V_6
R	Mean	6.1	11.3	6.9	3.5	5.4	11.5	17.2	11.8	14.9
	Range	1.0 / 13.8	3.0 / 20.0	0.2 / 17.2	1.0 / 7.5	0.5 / 13.6	4.1 / 28.5	2.5 / 33.2	5.0 / 19.5	4.0 / 27.0
	P_{90}	8.6	17.0	13.0	6.0	9.3	13.5	22.4	17.7	22.4
S	Mean	2.1	2.0	1.6	4.6	11.1	16.4	6.3	1.5	1.7
	Range	0.5 / 4.0	0.5 / 6.8	0.2 / 4.0	0.5 / 10.0	1.8 / 27.0	1.6 / 32.5	1.0 / 14.0	0.2 / 3.0	0.2 / 7.5
	P_{90}	4.8	5.5	3.0	7.3	16.4	23.8	10.5	2.6	2.2

DURATION (sec.

	Mean	Range	S.D.
P_{II}	0.085	0.072 / 0.103	0.028
P-R Seg. Lead II	0.045	0.020 / 0.078	0.017
P-R Int. Lead II	0.130	0.010 / 0.200	0.032
QRS	0.073	0.048 / 0.092	0.009
Q-T	0.300	0.228 / 0.372	0.025
Int. Def. V_1	0.018	0.010 / 0.030	0.005
Int. Def. V_6	0.033	0.017 / 0.048	0.006

RATIO

	Mean	Range	P_{90}
R:S in V_1	0.5	0.8 / 1.7	0.9
R:S in V_6	9.5	2.1 / 25.5	

TABLE 10
AMPLITUDE (mm.)

8 Years — 12 Years
(70 Subjects)

		I	II	III	V₁	V₆
P	Mean	0.8	1.1	0.7	0.9	
	Range	0.3 1.3	0.6 1.7	−0.3 1.8	0.1 2.3	
	P₉₀	1.2	1.6	1.2	1.9	
Q	Mean	0.5		1.3		1.1
	Range	0.1 2.8		0.1 4.0		0.1 3.7
	P₉₀	1.2		2.5		2.1

AMPLITUDE (mm.)

		I	II	III	V₃ᵣ	V₁	V₂	V₄	V₅	V₆
R	Mean	6.0	11.6	6.5	3.0	5.0	11.2	20.6	11.8	12.1
	Range	1.0 16.0	4.3 19.8	0.6 17.5	1.0 6.5	0.2 14.0	3.5 23.8	7.3 29.5	5.2 24.8	4.5 25.9
	P₉₀	9.3	16.7	11.7	4.4	8.8	13.2	21.9	17.8	19.8
S	Mean	1.4	2.3	2.6	5.2	11.4	16.3	6.3	2.1	1.5
	Range	0.3 4.2	0.2 7.2	0.2 8.3	0.2 16.0	3.0 28.5	3.7 30.0	0.2 14.0	0.2 10.2	0.2 4.2
	P₉₀	3.8	5.5	6.0	10.1	19.5	23.8	10.0	4.2	3.2

DURATION (sec.)

	Mean	Range	S.D.
P_II	0.089	0.050 0.124	0.018
P-R Seg. Lead II	0.051	0.022 0.088	0.028
P-R Int. Lead II	0.140	0.010 0.200	0.021
QRS	0.074	0.051 0.098	0.012
Q-T	0.340	0.260 0.400	0.011
Int. Def. V₁	0.019	0.010 0.032	0.006
Int. Def. V₆	0.033	0.018 0.045	0.003

RATIO

	Mean	Range	P₉₀
R:S in V₁	0.5	0.03 1.3	0.8
R:S in V₆	10.2	1.5 23.2	

TABLE 11
AMPLITUDE (mm.)

		I	II	III	V₁	V₆
P	Mean	0.9	1.2	0.7	0.9	
	Range	0.4 1.2	0.8 2.5	−0.2 1.9	0.1 2.4	
	P_{90}	1.0	1.9	1.6	1.8	
Q	Mean	0.4		1.1		1.1
	Range	0.1 2.2		0.3 3.0		0.2 3.2
	P_{90}	1.4		1.6		2.1

12 Years — 16 Years
(61 Subjects)

AMPLITUDE (mm.)

		I	II	III	V₁	V₂	V₄	V₅	V₆
R	Mean	6.4	12.1	7.4	3.2	7.6	13.6	16.2	13.7
	Range	1.5 16.2	5.0 22.3	0.6 20.0	0.2 13.0	3.2 20.5	1.2 34.0	5.0 30.0	4.8 27.0
	P_{90}	9.7	16.9	12.5	5.2	12.2	22.8	24.6	21.9
S	Mean	1.6	2.3	1.7	9.8	16.6	6.0	2.4	1.5
	Range	0.3 4.0	0.2 10.5	0.2 7.6	2.1 23.8	1.2 28.0	0.3 16.0	0.2 6.3	0.2 4.0
	P_{90}	3.0	4.8	5.8	15.4	25.0	12.8	4.3	2.8

DURATION (sec.)

	Mean	Range	S.D.
P_{II}	0.094	0.076 0.112	0.012
P-R Seg. Lead II	0.054	0.027 0.084	0.016
P-R Int. Lead II	0.148	0.088 0.200	0.026
QRS	0.078	0.058 0.100	0.011
Q-T	0.352	0.282 0.422	0.021
Int. Def. V₁	0.022	0.010 0.030	0.003
Int. Def. V₆	0.038	0.021 0.050	0.005

RATIO

	Mean	Range	P_{90}
R:S in V₁	0.4	0.02 1.4	0.7
R:S in V₆	10.0	2.0 28.0	

TABLE 12

AMPLITUDE (mm.)

		I	II	III	V$_1$	V$_6$
	Mean	0.9	1.2	0.7	0.8	
P	Range	0.5 / 1.4	0.7 / 2.4	−0.4 / 1.7	0.1 / 2.2	
	P$_{90}$	1.1	2.1	1.5	1.8	
	Mean	0.6		1.3		0.8
Q	Range	0.1 / 1.7		0.2 / 4.0		0.2 / 3.4
	P$_{90}$	1.1		2.3		1.6

16 Years — 20 Years
(66 Subjects)

AMPLITUDE (mm.)

		I	II	III	V$_1$	V$_2$	V$_4$	V$_5$	V$_6$
	Mean	7.6	12.0	6.8	2.7	6.6	14.0	14.7	12.9
R	Range	1.9 / 16.8	2.3 / 23.0	0.7 / 17.8	0.2 / 9.5	1.0 / 16.0	4.5 / 23.5	2.8 / 30.0	3.8 / 28.2
	P$_{90}$	11.2	16.2	12.9	4.7	12.8	20.5	21.3	18.4
	Mean	1.7	1.5	1.0	10.4	16.7	5.1	2.5	1.4
S	Range	0.2 / 4.8	0.2 / 6.0	0.2 / 9.8	3.6 / 23.4	8.0 / 28.0	0.4 / 11.6	0.2 / 7.0	0.2 / 5.0
	P$_{90}$	3.2	4.2	5.2	15.5	24.8	10.2	4.2	2.2

DURATION (sec.)

	Mean	Range	S.D.
P$_{II}$	0.090	0.076 / 0.118	0.014
P-R Seg. Lead II	0.052	0.025 / 0.082	0.015
P-R Int. Lead II	0.148	0.012 / 0.200	0.028
QRS	0.081	0.055 / 0.110	0.010
Q-T	0.362	0.324 / 0.420	0.020
Int. Def. V$_1$	0.021	0.005 / 0.040	0.004
Int. Def. V$_6$	0.038	0.020 / 0.055	0.005

RATIO

	Mean	Range	P$_{90}$
R:S in V$_1$	0.3	0.03 / 0.9	0.4
R:S in V$_6$	11.9	1.4 / 24.4	

TABLE 13
AMPLITUDE (mm.)

		I	II	III	V_1	V_6
P	Mean	0.8	1.2	0.8	0.8	
	Range	0.4 1.2	0.6 2.3	−0.3 1.4	0.2 2.2	
	P_{90}	1.0	2.1	1.1	1.7	
Q	Mean	0.3		1.7		1.4
	Range	0.1 3.0		0.2 4.0		0.2 4.0
	P_{90}	1.5		2.6		2.8

20 Years — 30 Years
(65 Subjects)

AMPLITUDE (mm.)

		I	II	III	V_1	V_2	V_4	V_5	V_6
R	Mean	5.9	13.1	8.6	3.7	6.9	16.6	17.0	12.8
	Range	1.3 12.8	5.0 24.0	1.3 24.1	0.1 9.0	2.2 13.2	4.3 30.8	5.0 30.0	5.0 25.5
	P_{90}	9.3	18.0	14.7	6.5	12.8	22.8	24.3	17.6
S	Mean	2.2	2.8	3.2	11.8	17.5	5.7	2.8	1.7
	Range	0.5 3.8	0.2 10.5	0.1 10.5	3.1 23.0	4.7 33.2	0.7 15.0	0.4 10.0	0.2 7.0
	P_{90}	3.0	5.2	6.0	18.0	25.2	13.2	4.6	3.0

DURATION (sec.)

	Mean	Range	S.D.
P_{II}	0.010	0.074 0.137	0.016
P-R Seg. Lead II	0.050	0.027 0.084	0.016
P-R Int. Lead II	0.151	0.010 0.200	0.021
QRS	0.081	0.080 0.110	0.010
Q-T	0.382	0.300 0.486	0.018
Int. Def. V_1	0.019	0.005 0.032	0.006
Int. Def. V_6	0.038	0.020 0.045	0.005

RATIO

	Mean	Range	P_{90}
R:S in V_1	0.4	0.01 1.3	0.6
R:S in V_6	10.5	2.4 23.2	

(288)

TABLE 14.—UPPER LIMITS OF THE NORMAL P–R INTERVALS (DURATION IN SECONDS)
(From Ashman and Hull)

Rate	Below 70	71–90	91–110	111–130	Above 130
Large adults	0.21	0.20	0.19	0.18	0.17
Small adults	0.20	0.19	0.18	0.17	0.16
Children, ages 14–17	0.19	0.18	0.17	0.16	0.15
Children, ages 7–13	0.18	0.17	0.16	0.15	0.14
Children, ages 1½–6	0.17	0.165	0.155	0.145	0.135
Children, ages 0–1½	0.16	0.15	0.145	0.135	0.125

TABLE 15.—DURATION OF QRS

(From Lüderitz, B.: Uber Beziehungen zwischen der Breite von QRS und erd Form des St Stuckes im menschlichen EKG (mit 7 Abb), Arch. f. Krcislaufforsch, 5, 223, 1939)

Duration of QRS sec.	Lead I per cent	Lead II per cent	Lead III per cent
0.06	3	0.8	1.8
0.07	20	19.0	17.0
0.08	46	43.0	43.0
0.09	13	25.0	24.0
0.10	4	10.0	10.0
0.11	1	1.0	1.8
0.12	0	0.8	0.4

TABLE 16.—UPPER LIMITS OF THE S–T SEGMENT IN LEAD WITH HIGHEST
T WAVE (DURATION IN SECONDS)
(From Ashman and Hull)

Rate	Men and children	Women
40	0.155	0.170
50	0.150	0.165
60	0.145	0.160
70	0.135	0.150
80	0.125	0.140
90	0.115	0.130
100	0.100	0.115
110	0.080	0.095
120	0.060	0.075
130	0.040	0.055
140	0.015	0.030
150	0.000	0.000

19

TABLE 17.—NORMAL VARIATIONS OF THE Q-T INTERVAL
(From Ashman and Hull and Lepeschkin)

Heart Rate (Min.)	Cycle Length (P–R interval) (Sec.)	Lower Limit (Sec.)	Mean (Sec.)		Upper Limit (Sec.)	
			Men & Child.	Women	Men & Child.	Women
40	1.50	0.42	0.45	0.46	0.49	0.50
43	1.40	0.39	0.44	0.45	0.48	0.49
46	1.30	0.38	0.43	0.44	0.47	0.48
48	1.25	0.37	0.42	0.43	0.46	0.47
50	1.20	0.36	0.41	0.43	0.45	0.46
52	1.15	0.35	0.41	0.42	0.45	0.46
55	1.10	0.34	0.40	0.41	0.44	0.45
57	1.05	0.34	0.39	0.40	0.43	0.44
60	1.00	0.33	0.39	0.40	0.42	0.43
63	0.95	0.32	0.38	0.39	0.41	0.42
67	0.90	0.31	0.37	0.38	0.40	0.41
71	0.85	0.31	0.36	0.37	0.38	0.41
75	0.80	0.30	0.35	0.36	0.38	0.39
80	0.75	0.29	0.34	0.35	0.37	0.38
86	0.70	0.28	0.33	0.34	0.36	0.37
93	0.65	0.28	0.32	0.33	0.35	0.36
100	0.60	0.27	0.31	0.32	0.34	0.35
109	0.55	0.26	0.30	0.31	0.33	0.33
120	0.50	0.25	0.28	0.29	0.31	0.32
133	0.45	0.24	0.27	0.28	0.29	0.30
150	0.40	0.23	0.25	0.26	0.28	0.28
172	0.35	0.22	0.23	0.24	0.26	0.26

TABLE 18.—DETERMINATION OF HEART RATE FROM CARDIAC CYCLE LENGTH
(Beats per minute)

Cycle Length (Sec.)	Heart Rate	Cycle Length (Sec.)	Heart Rate	Cycle Length (Sec.)	Heart Rate
0.04	1500	1.04	58	2.04	30
0.08	750	1.08	56	2.08	29
0.12	500	1.12	54	2.12	28
0.16	375	1.16	52	2.16	28
0.20	300	1.20	50	2.20	27
0.24	250	1.24	48	2.24	27
0.28	214	1.28	47	2.28	26
0.32	187	1.32	45	2.32	26
0.36	167	1.36	44	2.36	25
0.40	150	1.40	43	2.40	25
0.44	136	1.44	42	2.44	25
0.48	125	1.48	41	2.48	24
0.52	115	1.52	40	2.52	24
0.56	107	1.56	39	2.56	23
0.60	100	1.60	38	2.60	23
0.64	94	1.64	37	2.64	23
0.68	88	1.68	36	2.68	22
0.72	83	1.72	35	2.72	22
0.76	79	1.76	34	2.76	22
0.80	75	1.80	33	2.80	21
0.84	71	1.84	33	2.84	21
0.88	68	1.88	32	2.88	21
0.92	65	1.92	31	2.92	20
0.96	63	1.96	31	2.96	20
1.00	60	2.00	30	3.00	20

Electrocardiographic Criteria for the Diagnosis of Myocardial Disease

The diagnostic electrocardiographic criteria are presented in Lists I, II, and III, in order that the student may begin to acquaint himself with the relative significance of electrocardiographic observations. These lists are *not complete and cannot replace judgment, experience, and clinical correlating observations.* They are intended only to assist the beginner.

List I.—Definite Electrocardiographic Evidence of Myocardial Disease

1. Inversion, isoelectric, or extreme diphasicity of T_1, *not* due to digitalis or allied drugs, and few similar exceptions. The digitalis action may persist for three weeks after discontinuance of the drug.
2. Any degree of atrioventricular block (not caused by digitalis) or intraventricular block.
3. Clear deviation of the S–T level from the base line, as seen in infarction, angina pectoris, and pericarditis (page 115) (exclude digitalis and tachycardia).
4. Auricular flutter (almost always).
5. Auricular fibrillation (usually).
6. Ventricular fibrillation.
7. Ventricular paroxysmal tachycardia (usually).
8. Definite right axis deviation (110 degrees or more) with high P_1 and P_2 waves (usually).
9. Presence of two or three signs of Group II.
10. Alternation at slow or moderate ventricular rates (below 120). Exclude bigeminy (not always shown by the electrocardiogram).
11. Extreme left axis deviation with T_3 higher than T_1, and S_2 over 25 per cent of R_2.
12. Inverted T_4 (4V) in adults (exclude digitalis) and V_5 and V_6 if to the left of the transitional zone.
13. QRS, S–T, and T patterns of infarction in precordial leads.
14. Definite deviation of S–T due to infarction, angina pectoris, or pericarditis (exclude digitalis). (See page 115.)
15. Changing T waves not due to: (1) digitalis, (2) respiration, (3) Wolff-Parkinson-White syndrome, (4) position, etc.
16. Changing P–R interval (exclude digitalis and cardiac rate).
17. Extremely prolonged Q–T interval (Ca excluded).
18. Deep and usually wide Q_2 and Q_3 with inverted T_2 and T_3.
19. Axis of G normally does not lie more than 24 degrees to the right of the $\hat{A}_{QRS}$ axis.
20. Axis of G normally does not lie more than 35 degrees to the left of the $\hat{A}_{QRS}$ axis.
21. Certain other abnormalities in G.

List II.—Strongly Suggestive Electrocardiographic Evidence of Myocardial Disease

1. (*a*) Extremely low T waves in all leads, or in lead I (not due to polarization at the electrodes or to digitalization).
   (*b*) Extreme inversion of T_2 and T_3 isoelectric (exclude digitalis). Tracings must have been made with the subject in the supine position.

2. Less clear evidence of intraventricular block, such as slurring, Q or S waves present in all three leads, together with slightly prolonged QRS intervals, etc.
3. Deviation of S–T level from the base line in the standard leads (exclude digitalis and tachycardia), as discussed on page 104.
4. Extreme degrees of deviation of the QRS axis (page 99).
5. Extreme variability in the form of T (not respiratory) with moderate changes in cycle length.
6. Excessively low amplitude of the QRS complex in all leads (less than 5 millimeters).
7. Frequent multifocal or multiple ventricular premature beats or premature beats not eliminated by exercise. (This is considered by some to be definite evidence of myocardial disease.)
8. Increase of P_1 to *over* 1 millimeter and/or of P_2 to over 2.5 millimeters (needs confirmation).
9. Definite changes in the electrocardiogram occurring during the course of several months or a year.
10. Extreme left axis deviation with T_2 higher than T_1 and S_2 less than 25 per cent the amplitude of R_2.
11. Diphasic T in 4V and V_5 and V_6 if to the left of the transitional zone in adults (exclude digitalis).
12. Slightly prolonged Q–T interval.
13. Left axis deviation (fairly wide) with upright T_2.
14. Wide and notched P waves.
15. Abnormally shaped T_1.
16. Diphasic P (minus-plus type). This is questionable.

LIST III.—ELECTROCARDIOGRAPHIC SIGNS THAT SHOULD NOT IN THEMSELVES BE REGARDED AS EVIDENCE OF MYOCARDIAL DISEASE*

*This is an incomplete list.

1. Infrequent premature beats.
2. Inversion of T_3 in mild left axis deviation (transverse heart).
3. Slurring or notching in R or S of low amplitude, or at or near base, of a high R or S.
4. Moderate degres of deviation of the QRS axis.
5. Moderate decrease in amplitude of QRS.
6. Paroxysmal tachycardia of auricular or AV nodal origin.
7. Sinus arrhythmia.

LIST IV.—THE INTERPRETATION OF ELECTROCARDIOGRAMS—KEY FOR RECORDING

This suggested key has been found suitable for coding of electrocardiographic diagnoses and for writing quickly the interpretations of electrocardiograms. Only the number opposite each electrocardiographic observation is coded. By reference to this key chart, one can find the meaning of each number or certain electrocardiographic states from a "punch card" system of files. When an electrocardiogram is being read, it is only necessary to record the numbers, which can be translated later into a finished report.

Sinus Mechanisms:
1. Normal sinus rhythm.
2. Sinus tachycardia.

Sinus Mechanisms (Continued):
    3. Sinus bradychardia.
    4. Sinus arrhythmia.
    5. Sinus premature systole.
    6. Sinus arrest.

Auricular Mechanisms:
    7. Auricular premature systole.
    8. Auricular tachycardia.
    9. Auricular flutter.
  10. Auricular fibrillation.
  11. Wandering pacemaker.
  12. Impure flutter.
  13. Multiple premature contractions.
  14. Multifocal premature contractions.

Auriculoventricular (AV) Nodal Mechanisms:
  15. Auriculoventricular (AV) nodal premature systole.
  16. Auriculoventricular (AV) nodal rhythm.
  17. Auriculoventricular (AV) nodal tachycardia.
  18. Auriculoventricular (AV) nodal escape.
  19. Supraventricular tachycardia.

Ventricular Rhythms:
  20. Idioventricular rhythm.
  21. Ventricular escape.
  22. Ventricular premature systole: right, left, apical, basal or septal.
  23. Ventricular tachycardia.
  24. Ventricular fibrillation.
  25. Interpolated ventricular premature contractions.
  26. Multiple ventricular premature contractions.
  27. Multifocal ventricular premature contrations.
  28. Combination complexes.
  29. Retrograde conduction.
  30. Bigeminy.
  31. Trigeminy, etc.
  32. Electric alternation.
  33. Reciprocal beats.

Parasystole:
  34. Auriculoventricular (AV) dissociation with interference.

Mechanisms of Unknown Origin:
  35. Premature systole of unknown origin.
  36. Tachycardia of unknown origin.

Auriculoventricular Conduction:
  37. P–R interval normal.
  38. Incomplete AV block without dropped beats.
  39. Incomplete AV block with dropped beats.
  40. Complete AV block.
  41. Wenckebach phenomenon.

Intraventricular Conduction:
  42. QRS interval, normal.
  43. QRS interval, prolonged.

Intraventricular Conduction (Continued):
    44. Left bundle branch block.
    45. Right bundle branch block.
    46. Bundle branch block, unclassified.
    47. Bundle branch block, partial.
    48. False bundle branch block.
    49. Paroxysmal bundle branch block.

Mean Electric Axis of QRS:
    50. No deviation
    51. Left deviation
    52. Right deviation

P Wave:
    53. Normal voltage
    54. High voltage
    55. Low voltage
    56. Notched
    57. Diphasic
    58. Inverted
    59. Broad
    60. Isoelectric
    61. Auricular

QRS Group:
    62. Normal voltage
    63. Low voltage
    64. High voltage.
    65. Deep Q wave.
    66. Slurred, notched, or splintered.
    67. M or W shaped.
    68. S_1 wave present.

S–T (or R–T) Segment:
    69. Unusual elevation at origin.
    70. Unusual depression at origin.

T Wave:
    71. Normal voltage
    72. High voltage
    73. Low voltage
    74. Notched
    75. Diphasic
    76. Inverted
    77. Isoelectric
    78. Rightward deviation of T with leftward deviation of QRS.
    79. Leftward deviation of T with rightward deviation of QRS.
    80. Digitalis T wave.

Q–T Interval:
    81. Prolonged.

Q–T Patterns:
    82. Q_1T_1 pattern typical.
    83. Q_1T_1 pattern atypical.
    84. Q_3T_3 pattern typical.

Q–T Patterns (Continued):
  85. Q$_8$T$_8$ pattern atypical.
  86. Q–T pattern mixed (Q$_1$T$_8$, Q$_8$T$_1$).

Miscellaneous:
  87. U wave present.
  88. Artifacts.
  89. Unusual conditions not listed here.

Precordial Leads:
  90. V$_1$ to V$_6$.
  91. Esophageal lead.
  92. 4V—entire 4V lead normal.
  93. Abnormally low or absent R wave.
  94. S–T segment abnormally elevated.
  95. S–T segment abnormally depressed.
  96. Low T wave.
  97. Notched T wave.
  98. Isoelectric T wave.
  99. Diphasic T wave.
  100. Inverted T wave.
  101. Digitalis T wave.
  102. High T wave.
  103. IVB.
  104. IVR.
  105. Miscellaneous chest leads and observations not included above.

Interpretation:
  106. Normal electrocardiogram.
  107. Slightly suggestive electrocardiographic evidence of myocardial disease.
  108. Strongly suggestive electrocardiographic evidence of myocardial disease.
  109. Definite electrocardiographic evidence of myocardial disease.
  110. Compatible with posterior infarction.
  111. Posterior infarction.
  112. Compatible with anterior infarction.
  113. Anterior infarction.
  114. Lateral infarction.
  115. Septal infarction.

Serial Electrocardiograms:
  116. Serial electrocardiograms indicate significant change.
  117. Serial electrocardiograms show no significant change.
  118. Serial electrocardiograms indicate no significant change after exercise, or drugs, etc.
  119. Serial electrocardiograms indicate a significant change after exercises, or drugs, etc.

INDEX